How To Become A
Modern Viking

A Man's Guide To Unleashing The Warrior Within

Liam Gooding

How To Become A Modern Viking

A Man's Guide To Unleashing The Warrior Within

First Edition
(Edited 23rd June 2016)

Paperback Edition
ISBN-13: 978-1530623716
ISBN-10: 1530623715

Tomorrow's war is won during today's peace.

Tomorrow's winter is warmed from today's cut wood.

Tomorrow's maidens are seduced by today's hard work.

Contents

Viking Mindset 134

Now Go Viking! 213

Authors Notes 217

What's In This Book

Section Summaries

Viking Body

This section shows you how to work towards achieving a solid body as a man. You'll learn how important the connection is for a man's masculinity and his physical appearance.

This chapter is a combination of my own personal experience and research, combined with input from mentors and trainers who span Professional Bodybuilding, Strongman Competitors, Crossfit Coaches and MMA fighters.

However, this is not a book on fitness. It's a book on lifestyle.

This chapter explains where to find the balance between building a solid 6-pack and also knowing how to find time to enjoy a beer with the guys.

I will explain the techniques I've discovered to fit the huge nutritional requirements of a Viking with the pressures and stress of modern day life.

Viking Mindset

This section explores how to upgrade yourself from within. You'll learn the connection between your subconscious and your happiness and richness of experiences in life.

There is nothing in this chapter that I haven't developed from firsthand experience.

While you can purchase many books on Mindfulness, Neuro-Linguistic Programming (NLP) and self-hypnosis, I tend to find these books very "fluffy" and up in the clouds.

Instead, I present the techniques I've used to train my mind to be more courageous, to be more alpha and confident, and to be able to think like a Warlord and a King.

Going Viking

This section covers two follow up initiatives to continue your journey as a Modern Viking:

1. Brotherhood (Online community)
2. Tribes (Offline communities)

Both of which I believe to be an excellent way to grow the Modern Viking movement and improve the lives of more brothers and perhaps more importantly, to help you to take the next step after this book and stay on course through the tough times.

Not Just For "Manly Men"

Homosexual Men

I haven't watered down the fact that this book is about becoming a strong, masculine man in the very traditional and stereotypical sense, with a modern twist. This transformation is both a physical and psychological change, inspired by the strong characteristics and values of old Viking culture.

While I have a strong idea of how this helps heterosexual men in their personal and professional lives, I admit to not have all the answers on how becoming a Modern Viking can benefit homosexual men, especially very feminine homosexual men.

But, this is a book for men. *All men.*

I have many gay friends, and when I'm staying in San Francisco, around 50% of my male friends are gay (much to the suspicion of my straight male friends I'm sure!) The bottom line is, I'm a man comfortable in his sexuality. From a very young age, my father taught me that racism and homophobia were just scared and ignorant people thrashing out to hide their own lack of understanding.

So I choose my friends based on their values, ambition, value, character and positivity. Where they decide to stick their cock is irrelevant!

With this in mind, I think I have more access and perhaps more insight into the gay community than the average straight man.

However, I am still *nowhere near* close to a position to give advice on how a gay man might use my Modern Viking system. I don't know if a gay man can use this book to become more masculine to attract more men, or earn more respect in his workplace, or improve his relationships with his masculine friends.

Neither from my personal journey or through objective research, I'm just not informed enough on the matter.

The exception perhaps is the chapters on physical appearance and health - I believe that men are universally more appealing when we don't have doughy midsections, patchy skin and panting after 10 minutes of fucking.

My advice if you are reading this book as a gay or bisexual man is to take from the book the pieces that you feel will benefit you. Make your own judgments, and approach the book with an open mind and an ounce of mercy for me, the author. I mean well.

Nothing about my exploration of masculinity is exclusionary - I am not saying there is a *"right"* or a *"wrong"* way for a man to be. I believe Modern Viking masculinity is a choice - a choice open to straight, gay, bisexual or pansexual men. If you want to increase your masculinity modeled on ancient Vikings, then this book is for you. Who you choose to *pillage* and *plunder* with this knowledge is not my concern!

Women (Shield Maidens!)

I was writing a book for men. I knew I would talk to you, the reader, as if we were sitting sharing a few beers on the back patio, or perhaps over a BBQ on the beach or maybe on a drunk walk home after a fight together in a bar. I wanted to chat to one of my brothers, a guy I could relate to.

When I started this project, I couldn't imagine that women would be interested.

What I never expected was how many women would pre-order this book, follow my Instagram and Snapchat, and engage on the Facebook page.

In many cases I know women are taking an interest on behalf of their partners - and I find that great. This book after all is about helping men become better at being a man.

That means better husbands. Better boyfriends. Better fathers.

Another group of women are reading this for sheer curiosity about their counterparts - they want to get inside our heads as men. That's OK with me - if women knew the kind of men we Modern Vikings aspire to be, they'd be able to support it. They'd be able to figure out where they can fit into that journey. And they can learn how to spot one of those manly men when they're out looking for a man of their own!

With that said, I've still written the narrative of this book as if I'm chatting to a man. It's just easier, and speaks clearer to the other 75% of my readers who are men.

But you'll notice that there is no misogynistic or anti-feminism content in this book. Guess why?

Because I love women. Most men do.

Women and men are different (shock I know!). We have different dangly bits, we think differently, our biology is different, our brains are wired differently. Where I discuss the differences of women, please refrain from allowing any knee jerk "sexist" thoughts to cloud the room and cause you to miss the message.

Please read around masculine nouns and take from this book what you can. Certain chapters and notes around boosting testosterone are rather specific, as are the points on doing certain things to attract women (damn you ladies consume so much of our motivation!). But as most men will accept - you women are smarter than us, so I'm confident you'll be able to figure out which parts can apply and which parts to skip over.

If you're a Shield Maiden and you're particularly interested in how Modern Viking can apply to you, please connect with the Facebook page and be sure to drop me a message or an email. I plan to work on a specific 'Modern Shield Maidens' project (in collaboration) later in the year!

Vegetarians & Vegans

I make no apology for that fact that Vikings, and Modern Vikings, need to eat a lot of animal flesh. Fish, poultry, red meat... not only is it wonderfully delicious, it's a key component to testosterone release and protein intake in a man's diet.

If you're a vegetarian and you're reading this, you'll need to emphasize your dairy intake (particularly eggs) in order to get your protein intake. With that said, it won't be impossible.

If you're a vegan and reading this… wow I really don't have any answers. Without cheese, eggs, milk, fish and red meat, Vikings would not have ever existed. They would have been wiped out as soon as someone asked them to pick up a sword. Their weak undeveloped bones and their weak muscles would have been cut down by stronger men.

Being a Modern Viking is about the strong becoming stronger, and moving the weak out of their way.

With that said, and I've spoken to many awesome vegans during the research for this book, I really, really wish that animal welfare standards were in a better state right now. The mass production meat industry is quite simply, disgusting.

A Viking caught the fish he ate in his own nets. He salted and roasted the meat of deer and buck that he'd hunted with his own bow and arrow. He cooked the bacon from pigs that his whole family had fed, fattened and cared for, and they had said a prayer to thank the animal when it had been time for slaughter.

Vikings ate a lot of meat, fish and dairy products, but they did so with a healthy respect earned through hard work.

Unfortunately, the only way for a Modern Viking to get close to this and to try to remove their support for the awful standards in mass meat production is to always buy organic and free range. I know this carries an "elitist" label and price tag, but it should simply be *the price of meat.*

Not only is this meat free of antibiotics and pro-oestrogenic chemicals (yep - eating cheap meat kills your gains and gives you boobs), but the welfare standards around how the animals lived and were slaughtered are much better. You don't need to have a deep moral and ethical connection to animals, or watch some of the horror hidden-cam videos of some of these factories, to care.

You can focus on the fact that organic meat and free range dairy products are more nutritious, higher in protein, higher in omega-3, higher in creatine and taste so much better.

So if you're a vegan or vegetarian - I recommend you go and try some organic meat and free range eggs and then begin your journey as a Modern Viking![1]

---

[1] Of course I'm joking - do whatever the fuck you want! I won't preach that you should eat meat as long as you don't preach that I should stop eating meat

Introduction

My Story

I had everything. I owned a company valued at $6 million. I had cash in the bank. I had an amazing fiancée, who came from a good family, and every guy wanted to fuck her. She was literally perfect. I owned the perfect house ready to start a family. I was a tech genius. Life was perfect.

Except it wasn't.

I was depressed. I had achieved more than most men can hope for at my age, but I was intensely unhappy and unsatisfied.

I was insecure about my body. I wished I had more money, as much as my friends had. I wished I had sold my last company for millions like the guy I recently met at a Meetup. I wished my fiancée was nicer to me. I wished for a lot of things, based on whatever insecurity was bothering me that day. I couldn't feel happy with everything I had, only numb and envious about the things I *didn't have*.

I didn't know it at the time, but I had a huge hole inside me, and I'd tried to fill it with all of the wrong things. Nothing made me feel *really* happy, nothing made me feel confident, nothing made me feel secure.

Something was stopping me from being genuinely happy with my life. (And looking back, I really did have an amazing life!)

I remember that whenever I was alone for just an hour, I started to feel lonely. Anxious, fidgety. I needed to be with either a friend or my fiancée all of the time.

I spent more time obsessing over other people's startups or careers than I did my own. Rather than working on evening courses or reading books to improve myself, I spent the evening reading news sites, reading about other people's accomplishments rather than working on achieving my own.

I watched my friends approaching their 30's with hardened bodies. I saw them get pulled onto stages in clubs by groups of roaring bachelorette parties who wanted to see their abs. I watched from the sidelines and admitted the allure of a muscular man's body on a woman. All the time, I watched my body getting softer. The leanness and strength from my time training on the kickboxing squad for 6 days a week in University were gone. I started to leave a t-shirt on during sex. I started to get out of breath during sex. Eventually, I simply lost the drive to have sex entirely.

I would see my friends approaching girls for fun in bars, striking up conversations with women way out of their league. And the women became like putty in their hands.

I knew things didn't feel right. I knew this wasn't what a man was supposed to feel like each day. This was not the life of greatness I'd imagined for myself. And as you might expect, the cracks in my life started to appear.

Quite simply, it all fucked up. And there was no one to blame, but me.

However, that would be a pretty shitty and depressing end to a story, right? Don't worry, this is a book about change. A book to help men grab life by the balls and fucking run with it.

And that's exactly what I did!

I can tell you right now, I'm sitting here in a beautiful apartment, 10 minutes from the beach. I feel confident about my career. I'm confident in what my skills are, and what they aren't, and that's okay.

I'm sitting with my shirt off because I love how big and wide my body looks now. I look like a man. I feel great because tonight I had a date with a beautiful woman and it was awesome.

Don't misunderstand - this book isn't a guide to seduce women into your bed. It isn't a guide to get rich. And it isn't about how to live life as a location independent entrepreneur.

This book is about how to improve *you*, a modern man who has allowed life to turn him weak.

Too many people have told you that if you want the hot girlfriend or the flash car, all you need to do is attend a $2,000 one-day seminar, learn some system or some manipulative trick, and then *"go out into the world and take what's rightfully yours!"*

Sorry, but that's bullshit.

This book isn't about bullshit. It isn't about short cuts, tricks, or manipulations.

It's a story of how I discovered my inner strength, my inner warrior, and focussed on me. I looked at some of the strongest male figures history provided, the Vikings, and took inspiration.

I took a step backwards, and forgot about all of the external shit in life that I was supposed to desire. I stopped chasing women. I stopped worrying about other people, their girlfriends, their jobs, their houses or their flashy cars.

I just looked at *myself* and thought, *"How the fuck am I going to make ME more awesome?"*

Who Were The Vikings?

The Vikings were Scandinavian farmers and fisherman who thought bigger. They sailed forth from Sweden, Denmark and Norway and discovered rich lands filled with treasure, guarded by weak men.

And as is the way of man, the strong take from the weak.

Vikings ventured out as pirates and conquered territory across northern Europe. They became notorious throughout Europe for their brutal efficiency, excellent battle tactics and fierce, near primal, courage in battle.

Viking Raids

Vikings are one of the groups of people in history we know so little about because we mostly only have the records from one side - the people who they attacked. While Vikings did have a basic written language system and a Runic alphabet, most Vikings could not read or write, and usually only one or two of the elders and healers/shaman in the village would know how to read and write.

Instead, most of the history of Vikings was recorded by Christian priests - who were usually on the pointy end of Viking swords. As you can imagine, this perspective is likely responsible for the bias in the descriptions of the Viking raiders brutality, savagery and cold efficiency.

Vikings first raided outside of Scandinavia in the latter half of the 8th century, raiding at Lindisfarne Monastery, England in the year 793[2]. Raiding monasteries would continue to be a favourite pastime of the Vikings for the decades that followed - they were undefended and held rich plunder.

As time went on, Viking raids became more common across Britain and Europe.

In 837, a cleric in Aachen, Germany observed: *"the Northmen at this time fell on Frisia with their usual surprise attack"* [3] [4].

From the 840's, Vikings began to winter in enemy territory rather than return with their plunder to Scandinavia. They would build fortified encampments, making raids the following year even easier and, in many instances, prompting the local monarchies to pay huge sums of ransom for the Vikings to leave.

Eventually, Vikings started to ask for land in payment instead of gold and silver. Treaties and oaths were formed, tied in marriage between Anglo-Saxon and Viking families. This trend continued across Ireland and Northern France (where the Vikings , under Rollo[5], would eventually colonise and establish the Duchy of Normandy).

Viking raids were incredibly far reaching, stretching across most of Northern Europe, and even reaching as far as Canada and Africa!

---

[2] https://www.lindisfarne.org.uk/793/

[3] "The Annals Of St-Bertin", *Janet Laughland Nelson*. https://books.google.com/books?isbn=0719034256

[4] http://www.britannica.com/place/Frisia

[5] Brink, Stefan, and Neil S. Price. *"The Duchy Of Normandy." The Viking World.* London: Routledge, 2008

Vikings Were Not Good Men

As Pagans invading a Christian population, Vikings were perceived as savages and Godless heathens. They raided without mercy, sacking villages and killing anyone in their way. They were also known for capturing their enemies for use as slaves when space in their ships allowed.

The phrase *'Rape, pillage and plunder'* is quite historically accurate, even if the history was recorded almost entirely by their victims.

Just as with any historical tribe of people, a lot of things about the Vikings are barbaric and despicable by today's modern societal standards. Slavery. Rape. Conquest. These aren't great moral ideals (but certainly not exclusive to Vikings).

But we are not looking at Vikings to learn how to become *good men*. As Jack Donavan discusses in *'The Way Of Men'*, we want to become *good at being men*. As you'll see in subsequent chapters, the two goals are very different and while the Vikings weren't exactly the best at *being good men*, they were great at *being men!*

We Stopped Being Real Men

The two most common reasons that men become soft, weak and insecure are:

1. Because somewhere along the way, society encouraged men to believe that it was okay to not "be a real man"
2. Because a woman in your life made you think it was okay to not "be a real man"

Society Made Men Soft

We often discuss "being a man" or a "real man" in the context of manly virtues. Ask random people to describe characteristics of a virtuous man and they will say things such as "strength, courage, honor, kindness, compassion, morality".

Virtues originates from the latin *'virtus'* from *'vir'* meaning man. The Romans used *'virtus'* to refer specifically to martial accomplishments on the battlefield. To say a man had virtue was to say he had shown valor, bravery, strength and courage on the battlefield.

However, the borders of Rome expanded. Men were left inside the peaceful territories without the fires of battle to earn *virtus*, so the definition and use expanded to include social and political values.

Suddenly, the attainment of virtue became less about physical strength or courage, and more about moral conduct within society. A physically soft and weak man could still be a good man.

What a shame.

Indeed, our borders are not being ravaged by barbaric men, eager to take what we have, by strength of spear and axe. Being a strong and courageous man does not offer the same group survival benefits (or requirement!) like it once did. With the exception of courageous women and men who choose to enlist in the military, police force of fire service, there are very few opportunities or requirements today to run into a high risk situation in the name of *virtus*.

But we should not forget - so much of our masculinity is tied to this heritage. Is it any surprise that as a man allows himself to become physically weak, his mindset becomes weak? His biological appeal to a women becomes weak? The respect he receives from other men, who are biologically wired to respect and admire strong men, also falls?

When we allow society to make us weak, to give us an excuse, a free-pass to softness, we invite weakness and softness into all aspects of our lives and relationships.

Your Woman Made You Soft

Most groups of friends have heard and made the jokes:

- "She owns his balls now!"
- "She wears the trousers now!"
- "He was castrated as soon as he put that ring on her finger!"

Misguided feminists (as in, the *'feminists'* who are not feminists but in fact looking for angry fuel to burn a fire of hate against men) will see these phrases and latch onto them with a vigor and anger to check the Gods! *"Empty sexist comments from misogynistic pigs!"*

However, the origin of these jokes is often legitimate.

Too many men allow themselves to become soft and weak when they fall in love. Comfort, contentment and security allow a man to lower his guard. His biological imperatives to stay strong and sharp are diminished - and why would they not be?

He has a beautiful woman - biologically speaking, this fulfils his urge to procreate. If he also has a home and stable career, he also has the security required to relax. His borders are safe and he can sheathe his sword in a scabbard each night.

Whereas a woman, who will have stronger "nest building" instincts, will maintain her strength, or even increase it. Organizing the family, the home and her own career, she was never driven by a masculine need to fight or protect.

Standing by the side of this female strength, too many men decide to take a back seat. To become weak. To become comfortable.

And in the process, allow themselves to become a different man than the one his woman fell in love with. A different man than the one his boss hired. A different man than his friends respected.

Have You Lost Your Way?

Are you the guy who hangs out at the fringes of the group, while your more confident and charismatic friends chat up a group of beautiful women?

Are you the guy who silently complies when your boss chooses you to stay an extra 2 hours and man the phones, while the rest of the team go for an early beer?

Are you the guy who quietly grumbles to himself when someone cuts in line at the store - and looks down at your shoes when the person turns around to stare at you and intimidate you even further?

Are you the guy who meekly tells your wife that you're heading to bed alone, leaving her behind on the sofa watching her drama while she chats to her girl friend on the phone?

Are you the guy who spends his entire pay check every week on designer clothes so that you can hang out in the background of pretentious wine bars, nursing your 2008 Rioja and fidgeting with your phone every 5 minutes?

Are you the guy buying $40 cocktails for beautiful women in trendy lounges, only for them to walk away from the bar to their table giggling as they go?

Are you the guy who can't have sex for longer than 15 minutes because you're out of breath?

Are you the guy spending 75% of your monthly income on lease payments for a sports car that you can hardly afford the gas for?

Are you the guy wearing his t-shirt at the beach? Or worse, wearing his t-shirt during sex with the lights off?

Are you the guy simply watching the beautiful woman in the bar, nervously fidgeting each time she smiles over at you, until eventually she pays her tab and leaves alone?

Are you the guy living in a 2,000 sq. ft *'party apartment'* that gets trashed every weekend by your 'friends'?

Are you the guy walking down the street hunched over, looking down, scared to make eye contact with anyone you walk past? Especially the beautiful woman who just smiled at you over her coffee?

Are you the guy who girls describe to their friends as *"seems like a nice guy with a great personality, good boyfriend material"* before they swipe left and then scream *"Ooooh yes!"* at the huge armed, wide shouldered and shredded abs guy on the next profile?

Are you the guy spending more time reading blogs and watching Youtube videos of awesome people, than you are actually spending trying to become more awesome?

You might read most of these questions with your ego and pride set to maximum, and say *"No way - that's not me!"* and if that's the case, then congratulations! You're a confident, self-assured, socially and physically strong man! Maybe you're already a Modern Viking and you just didn't know it?

But chances are that at least one of those resonated with you.

We rush things. We try to get the girl before we've made ourselves into someone who can add value to the girl's life. We try to get the lifestyle before we've accumulated the income to sustain it. We try to buy status before we've earned it.

Sometimes this happens as part of a regression - we've been confident and secure in the past, but a life event happens that causes us to panic and start acting from a place of desperation and fear. A divorce, a redundancy, house foreclosure, a breakup, weight gain.

Other times, we've just known no other way. Your parents lived beyond their means. Your friends are awkward around women. Your colleagues all rent apartments they can't afford. You've never believed in investing your money into *the system*.

Weakness, softness, over exuberance, weak friends, insecurity, low-self-esteem… these are enemies of the Modern Viking.

Our goal is to build a strong foundation in ourselves so that we can build outwards and attract these things naturally and honestly, and keep them once we have them.

When we create a strong version of ourselves, we attract other strong men. And once we have strong men by our side and the ambition and strength to do something with that strength, we can go out into the world and pillage and plunder from all of the weak and pathetic men who are holding all the gold and women! The strong take from the weak!

Becoming A Modern Viking

You want to be more masculine so that you can get more from life. More wealth. More sex. More love. More success. More excitement.

How are you going to get there? What are the qualities you want to build in yourself? What exactly is a Modern Viking?

I created the concept of a Modern Viking to become an ideal that a man could build towards. I created it for myself, for my own journey, but part of my own journey was that I wanted to inspire and help other men along their own path too.

So here's how I see it.

the way of the Modern Viking is the way a Viking would live today if he'd adapted to modern civilization. If modern knowledge, security and resources were at his disposal, but he still had the inner strength, courage and attitudes that had been forged into him by his Viking culture.

I personally created this concept of a Modern Viking - and I am neither a University PhD Historian, an Olympic Weightlifter or a Doctor of Psychology.

But I believe I've put together a great formula through my own experience, trial and error, and a lot of research!

It takes inspiration from Viking and Norse culture, but it has little to do with battle re-enactment or practicing Norse religion (Asatru). You don't need to listen to Viking Thrash Metal and you don't need to wear black t-shirts depicting Odin's Mark.

Instead, you'll be inspired by the strength and masculinity of the Vikings. By their culture of brotherhood. By their focus on self improvement. By their desire to be the best trained warriors on the battlefield.

Once you become a Modern Viking, you will:

- Be the Alpha male of most situations
- Be physically muscular, stronger and healthier
- Have strong, confident posture
- Be confident and self-assured in your everyday life
- Be confident and natural when flirting with women
- Have a strong tribe who make you better and more successful
- Understand the value and benefits of Brotherhood
- Be willing to go into frightening situations and understand how to handle your fear and understand risk-reward
- Understand how to dress to project a strong masculine image

Some of these may not immediately appeal to you - however my own experience with becoming a Modern Viking was that the more I achieved and progressed, the more I wanted to dive in.

For example, my immediate concern was how to look better. It started as a simple theory that my unhappiness and depression came from the fact that I didn't look attractive to women anymore.

I didn't care that the health improvement would also upgrade my sex life, the quality of my relationships with friends and women, or my professional career.

But once I started to look and feel like a Viking, I became more interested in how an increased physical and mental masculinity improved other aspects of my life, and I loved it!

I noticed how my new self-assuredness and health positively affected my productivity and career - my energy levels were higher and my passion for leadership increased. I investigated the world of PUA ('Pick Up Artists') and realised how hard many of these guys had to work on their *tricks* and *deceitful manipulations* to compensate for their small skinny bodies and awkward postures.

I learned how much my long-term health, ability to fight disease, and even survive cancer, were improved by having increased muscle mass. I started to notice which friendships were conducive to my daily motivation and positivity, and which were a source of negativity or complacency.

For this reason, I've broken down the process of becoming a Modern Viking into a system that works well as a natural progression. As you move through each of these steps, your motivation for the process will increase. You'll start receiving positive feedback on your transformation within a few weeks - this encouragement is important to keep your motivation levels high, especially during the times when it will be hard work.

Becoming a Modern Viking involves working on these two key components:

1. A Viking Body
2. A Viking Mindset

This book may seem like a series of things you just need to *"Do"* and then your journey is complete. But life is not that simple or linear.

You will for example, begin to notice huge gains in confidence after only 3 months of working on your physical self. You might meet a new girl in a bar thanks to your slightly improved body and confidence. Or you might get a small promotion at work.

But this does not mean that you stop working on your body! That's probably the most common reason why guys end up with never achieving the body, love life or career they wanted!

Becoming a Modern Viking is not about achieving mediocracy or average life. We're striving for greatness - for something that other men will look upon and dream of! The beautiful and loving wife and family, the big house, the fast car... whatever it is that's important to you and you want to achieve, all needs to be acquired slowly. Acquire them on a solid foundation built on a better, stronger you. Modern Vikings don't sprint and chase after wealth and women - they build a version of themselves that naturally attracts wealth and women!

Your journey is not complete after simply reading this book either. Building a great physique takes years. Building a rock solid mindset can take just as long, if not longer.

For this reason, I have created a follow-up program called *Modern Viking: Brotherhood* where you can share your journey with likeminded men who have all committed to a life transformation.

You can explore Brotherhood on the website here:

http://liamgooding.com/brotherhood

Brotherhood is a membership-supported community. Modern Vikings worldwide can chat and support each other, hold each other accountable to goals, and can share stories and tips along the way.

And because it runs on mobile as a lightweight private chat app, there is also plenty of banter and fun in there too!

As a private group of the most committed Modern Vikings, Brotherhood is also the early development lab for new ideas, guides and resources that I create for the community.

I encourage you to take a look after reading this book and of course, contact me with any questions or suggestions you may have:

Email me: hello@liamgooding.com

Viking Body

Why Build A Viking Body

The first stage on your Modern Viking transformation is to create a body that looks masculine, can endure the rigors and pressures of true masculine life, and is the sort of body that women are biologically attracted to.

It's impossible for us to aspire towards a greater sense of masculinity; to a higher level of manliness internally; to becoming Vikings, without building the masculine body that millions of years of evolution has perfected.

Men are stronger than women. Men have more muscle mass than women. Men are typically taller than women. Anyone who pretends to ignore these simple facts from under a banner of sexual equality is stupid.

Whether you are conscious of it or not, when you see two men side by side and one is muscular and the other is not, you assume the more muscular man is the most masculine, i.e., he is further away from the body shape and composition of a woman. By simple logic then, it's clear to see that one of the quickest ways to achieve a greater perception of masculinity would be to increase your muscle mass (you aren't going to get taller anytime soon I'm afraid!)

By looking the part, you begin to feel the part.

Becoming a Modern Viking means building your body to be what it was meant to be. A body to survive the harsh realities of life. A body with the endurance and stamina to hunt down and kill wild animals so that you can eat them. A body with the strength to build a sturdy and resilient shelter for your mate and offspring. A body with the raw power and agility to triumph in the ultimate physical test of killing other men who threaten to take your resources.

Men and women are hardwired to respect these qualities in a man because it's how we've survived for thousands of years. Even though modern society doesn't threaten you with the same physical dangers and tests, you still have those same wire inside of you and your body still functions optimally when it's built this way.

When Vikings landed in England, they were larger, stronger and better trained than most Anglo-Saxon soldiers they came up against. Multiple battle accounts describe men who *"stood a head taller and a half breadth wider than their foes"*. There is little you can do to become taller, however by allowing your body to grow the largest muscular build it was destined to have, you become closer to being a Modern Viking.

Gaining Respect From Men

Whether we like to admit it or not, we respect other men who are big and muscular. We respect their manliness. We respect their authority when they speak. Even if we don't like the person, we respect them.

Respect based on physical appearance makes sense from a Darwinistic point of view - if a man looks like he will be valuable to the tribe, he probably will be. It's rare that a man would be physically muscular but useless at erecting a shelter, or useless at hunting or fighting. These triggers are still within us and they transfer to modern life.

If you work in an office, think about how you instinctively feel about the guys who are overweight and out of shape. When you see their large trousers hanging underneath their huge guts, their big sweat stains, their fat fingers cramming potato chips into their mouth at their desk. The wheezing as their climb the 3 flights of stairs while grumbling that the elevator is out of order. Depending on how strong your fear of *"political correctness"* is - you probably think this person is weak.

Because fat guys with no muscle mass are weak.

And likewise, think about the skinny, frail looking guys in your office. The ones who hunch their tiny feminine shoulders in when they walk. Who's size Extra-Small shirts hang off their skeletal frame like a female runway model. Who need to ask for help to move their PC monitor. You probably don't respect this guy much, and think he's weak.

Because skinny guys with no muscle mass are weak.

Both the fat guy with no stamina and the skinny guy with no strength would be cut down on the battlefield within the first few minutes. Perhaps the fat guy might prove a bit more useful in the shield wall, but within a few minutes his arm would tire and his huge bulk would go from 'advantage' to 'burden'. The skinny guy would probably have gone down in the first charge, or maybe he slipped around with a knife for a while (like Loki the trickster) before eventually getting overwhelmed.

Being skinny and weak, or being fat and weak inherently makes people lose respect for you. You can be the nicest guy in the office, or the smartest guy, or the funniest guy, but people will still not respect you *as much* as if you were muscular and (moderately) lean.

Think about the guy who goes to the gym 3-4 days a week. Who eats okay. I don't mean the "health freak" who's always talking about being Paleo, because that guy is usually irritating. But think about the guy who stands tall when he walks around the office, who looks like he could move furniture without effort, who looks like he could pick up the blonde receptionist and carry her to his office!

Whether you are aware of it or not, you respect that guy more. You subconsciously listen to him with more reverence. He has more gravitas when he enters the room.

Commanding respect involves many factors, and I'm not saying that someone fat has no respect, or that someone muscular has the most respect. But it's guaranteed that for the *same person*, you would respect them more if they were physically larger in a muscular way.

Take a hard look at yourself, and be honest. I'm not here to coddle you. Do you think you're missing out on an opportunity to gain respect from people because of the way you look?

As a Modern Viking we want to gain the maximum respect from people around us. Our families, friends, sexual partners, colleagues, or simply the people we meet in our daily lives.

Living Longer, Living Better

You hear all the time that if you workout at the gym and follow a 'healthy diet', you'll be 'healthier'. Gyms throw this at you. Zumba classes throw this at you. Whole Foods throws this at you complete with a 50% markup on your bag of 'healthier' carrots.

But 'being healthier' is an extremely general and usually intangible concept for most people to grab on to.

However, when I tell you about building a Viking Body, I'm telling you that you will gain more muscle mass. You will get stronger. You will get your body fat in check. You will have increased levels of free testosterone. Your anxiety and stress levels will be lowered.

But best of all, you are scientifically proven to live longer. You will have an increased chance of surviving cancer and other serious disease. You will even have a higher chance to survive serious accidents.

There is a direct correlation, from multiple studies, showing that if a man holds more muscle mass then he will literally win The Game of Life or Death more often.

Building a Viking Body and sticking to your disciplined diet isn't selfish - sure you're going to look amazing and feel amazing. But you can walk into this process knowing that your wife will have a healthy husband for longer. Your children will have an active father for longer. You'll have more time to do more pillaging and plundering!

Putting Your Body First

Modern Viking is an entire lifestyle upgrade, not a workout routine. However, there's a lot of good reasons why we get started on the body first:

1. It requires no one else but yourself

2. An intense fitness program will give you more energy, more endorphins and crucially, more testosterone

3. A masculine physique will make you naturally more confident in groups

4. You'll see almost immediate results, which is very important for motivation through the more difficult stages of becoming a Modern Viking

5. Your physical transformation will shut down any haters who are themselves talking from a place of their own jealousy and insecurity

6. You'll build strong self-discipline, which you'll notice will transfer to other areas of your transformation

It Requires Only Yourself

Transforming your Viking Body is something you can simply wake up and start doing. You don't need to start interacting with the friends and family in your life differently. You don't need to start interacting with the women you're romantically pursuing differently. There are no other variables or obstacles (i.e., She really does have a boyfriend, your boss really doesn't have budget, your wife really does have a headache , etc.)

You simply need to build the knowledge, build the habits, and start grinding.

Increased Energy

A full lifestyle upgrade is a hard and difficult journey on its own, even without adding the pressures of regular life too.

You might be looking to a Modern Viking transformation to find strength during a divorce, breakup, depression... or simply because life has burned you out.

When you're facing something like this, one of the most valuable resources you need is energy. Willpower. Focus. It has many names, but it's the force that pulls you out of bed at 6.30am instead of 10.30am. It's the reason you don't turn on the TV at 7pm, and instead you get your ass in a cold shower and then head out to that Meetup. It's the driving force that pushes you back into the gym for the 5th day that week, despite the fact your legs can barely operate the car pedals.

Working out gives you more energy. More endorphins (i.e., happy juice for your brain). More testosterone.

And all of these things are what we want to be happy men. We need to resist the urge to do nothing. The temptations of modern life that made us weak and soft. The temptation to sit up at night stalking your ex's Facebook profile while using your tears as lube.

Increased Confidence In Groups

As we'll discuss in more detail later, we are extremely visual in judging someone. We can learn to appreciate the personality of someone after meeting them, however during the first moments when we see someone, we form a first impression of them.

This is true of women, who yes, despite all they proudly say to the contrary, would rather fuck a man with a 6 pack than one without one.

But it's especially true of men. Men are by far the most visually driven of the 2 genders. This is why you still want to fuck stupid, amoral and shallow women - because they also happen to have a beautiful face, big tits and a round ass. This is not me being shallow - this is just science.

What many men overlook though is that this same visual mindset applies to men judging men too. Other guys judge you based on your appearance, your physical body shape, how you dress, how you stand, how you walk, how you sit.

If you look like you're strong; able to add to the collective strength of the tribe and defend their resources from other attackers, they will respect you as a brother in arms. A shield wall is built entirely on the strength of the men to your sides and the man behind you!

If you have low body fat, they'll respect your ability for self-discipline. You're proving that you aren't gluttonous, you can control your own desire to over-consume resources and you won't damage the survival chances of the whole group.

If you dress well, they'll know you're concerned about the social status of the whole group. You want to reflect well on the group, you know how to attract other females into the group - an asset which naturally benefits everyone.

If you improve your Viking Body, you'll increase your respect from the group and find it much easier to feel more confident in that group. With confidence, you'll feel more relaxed with talking and demonstrating your other qualities and value as a man.

Seeing Results Provides Motivation

If you follow the advice and physical program in Modern Viking, you'll start to see results within weeks.

I know because I did. And other guys who have followed my advice have seen immediate results too. This is important because men are impatient. We push a rock, we expect it to roll. We go hunting, we expect to eat meat. When we put effort and energy into something and don't see results from it pretty soon, we drop it.

How many bullshit exercise gadgets do you have laying around your home? The reason you stopped using your 'Abs Masturbator' wasn't because you felt like an idiot using it (plenty of weightlifting exercises look stupid!) but because after 2 weeks of following the program to the letter, nothing improved.

Modern Viking was designed for men only. The fitness and diet industry is over 80% female, so most of the advice out there is aimed at women because that's where the money is.

But men have a unique biology. Our bodies want to be stronger. Our bodies want to look a particular shape. Every man's body wants to be a strong and powerful machine of muscle mass designed to excel at protecting, fighting, and fucking!

This means when you follow the testosterone boosting, muscle-mass building, body-fat cutting diet and lifestyle of Modern Viking, you'll see pretty much immediate results.

Results that keep you motivated to keep pushing.

Your Transformation Will Shut Down Haters

You need to ignore the haters and negative people for optimal results in Modern Viking. But they're going to find ways to get through. Jealous friends are going to mock you obsession with fitness. Party friends are going to hate that you don't go out clubbing 3 nights a week anymore. Your ex is still going to send you shitty texts. (My ex was kind enough to send me photos of her in bed with various men, or the occasional photo of a ripped guy with the simple text "Just fucked him").

There will be haters. Some more extreme than others. Some from a position of jealousy or bitterness. Their own insecurities. Some who just want their relaxed, beer-bellied buddy back.

But in my experience, nothing shuts down all of these haters better than when they see that first shot of you looking like a beast. That first time they see you walking tall, looking big, and catching eyes of every girl in the bar as you walk over to them.

In some cases, they'll just shut up and disappear and leave you to your own positive journey without them. In other cases, they'll change their opinion and gain respect for you. Or in some cases, they might ask if you want to go on a date!

Obviously, there is still much more work for you to do before you're immune to the bullshit and negativity of these people. They'll still have power and influence over you until you're fully transformed into a Modern Viking. But when they see you becoming a beast, they'll be forced to respect your journey.

Self-Discipline

Crafting the Modern Viking physique is going to require a strong self-discipline. Which you probably don't have right now. Self-discipline is one of the most important values to maintain to make the transformation successful.

When a Viking woke up at 6am, he went out and fed the animals with his son, he hauled in nets, he repaired the roof leak from the previous night, he practiced swordsmanship, he drilled shield formations with his crew... and maybe then he went to eat lunch!

Working on a huge self transformation will require waking up and sticking to a program for the full day - it will require big and painful changes which will not be pleasant.

Learning to attack those difficult tasks starts with learning to attack the doughy piece of shit you call your body. You need to grind your ass - 4 to 6 days a week - if you're following the Modern Viking workout program. There are no excuses, there are no "cheat days". When you cheat, you cheat yourself; you give yourself a pass.

You've already given yourself enough passes. That's what got you into this shit. Just one more donut. Just one more beer. Just one more slice of pizza. It's always *just one more*.

The amazing thing, and I saw this with my own journey, was once I'd accepted the pain, the difficulty, the inconvenience of working out in the gym every day in the week, suddenly adding other small changes wasn't hard.

When asked about his 'almost military' discipline in his personal life, from eating to a timed schedule no matter where he was or what he was doing, to having an immaculately clean and tidy apartment, Arnold Schwarzenegger once said *"Bodybuilding was a good way of introducing more discipline and control into the rest of your life"*.

Reading one book a week? No problem. Attending one new networking event a week, no sweat. Compared to leg day, that's nothing.

When we look at someone with a great physique, particularly in office environments, we subconsciously judge that person as self disciplined. That's no mistake. Getting to a strong masculine physique takes discipline. Not the kind of "dust eating, liquid pooping, endless starving" type discipline of bullshit diets in women's magazines. In fact one of the most fun things about a Modern Viking body transformation is the diet! However, the work, the grind, the commitment to "embracing the suck" and putting your body as the top priority each week, that takes a lot of self discipline.

Increased Raw Sexual Connection

When you're with a woman, whether it's a girl for a casual one night stand or a your wife of 20 years, we all know that a woman's attraction is a complex equation of many variables.

Comfort. Excitement. Security (i.e., are you rich?). Lust. Intrigue. Infatuation. Fantasy…

There are many reasons why a woman might choose to kiss, or be kissed by, you. There are many reasons why she might choose to give you a blow job. There are many reasons why she might choose to have sex with you.

But at the moment when you're fully undressed, naked, sweaty, and resting your sword deep in her sheath, there's only one thing at play. Your raw physical connection.

Some women might fuck you because you drive a Lamborghini. Other women might fuck you because they love you; because you make them feel safe and wanted.

But once they start fucking you, and you're in the middle of plundering her valuables, we're down to the same physical connection that humans have had for thousands of years. With the exception of cultural/fashion preferences of how you both might trim your bushes, nothing has changed about the way we fuck. For thousands of years.

And unsurprisingly, when you start to build yourself the strong, physical body of a man as you were meant to be - a strong, wide backed, muscular man - you'll find you fuck a lot better.

Trust me.

The woman currently providing an anvil for your Thor's Hammer will respond differently to you. More primal, more animalistic. She'll run her hands over your wide shoulders, over your bulging chest, and your thick biceps. Multiple studies also support a theory that an increase in your sexual pheromones (Androstenone and Androstadienone) caused by increased testosterone levels will also make her hornier for you.

I keep coming back to the issue of motivation because we aren't trying to run a 30 day "eat and shit only wheatgrass and lemonade" fad diet. This is not a painful bootcamp and once it's over, you can relax again.

Modern Viking is an entire life transformation and that requires dedication and motivation to stick to it.

And that gets much easier when the sex with your casual partners, or your girlfriend, or your wife (or all 3!) becomes better. More rewarding, more exciting, more masculinizing.

Getting Bigger

One of the defining principles about the Modern Viking program is size. Becoming a Viking means building muscle; getting big. Forget all the bullshit about "toning up" or "slimming down" or "turning fat into muscle" or whatever other bullshit phrases small guys say.

Our goal is to look big. To look "manly". That means building a wide and thick back. Large rounded shoulders. Thick biceps and triceps. A large panelled chest. Strong and powerful abs and obliques (even though it's very likely they won't show through the fat on your abdomen - which is totally OK).

You might be fat big right now, or "fat-skinny" (tiny arms but a big beer gut), or just skinny. Regardless of where you are right now, everything about following the Modern Viking program is designed to add more muscle mass and more size, but with a controlled body fat percentage.

Viking Exercise Principles

Principles Before Spreadsheets

Unlike 99% of workout books or guides out there, Modern Viking isn't a fixed program or routine. This isn't a 90 day crash course workout program that will burn you out, bend and break you and (likely) make you quit. Trying to take on a sudden and fixed program just doesn't work, and it's why there's such a booming fitness industry around these programs.

So many people start them - buy the book, buy the DVDs, buy the $100 velcro straps… and then try and follow an intense and impractical program for 30 days with no flexibility. Most people fail. They stay fat, skinny, or both, and wait a few months until another life event (birthday, new year, breakup) gives them another kick towards buying into the next fitness fad program.

I know this cycle because I'd repeated it myself many times. I've bought the ab roller and DVD. I've bought the TRX bands. I've bought the workout DVD boxsets.

When I started to create the Modern Viking program for myself, I knew that the simple and pragmatic program I would actually commit to would be 10 times more effective than the intense but complicated program that I would quit.

Instead of a fixed plan, a fixed routine, a quirky gimmick, I built Modern Viking around a set of principles and guidelines. When you learn these guidelines and build them into your lifestyle, you can actually "live" the life of a Modern Viking and the Viking body will follow.

That's why I called this book 'How To *Become* A Modern Viking' - because it becomes a way of life for you, slowly. You don't need to print out excel spreadsheets and live your life on the scales. And it's so much more than a workout routine.

At its essence, training to become a Modern Viking comes down to 3 key principles:

1. Lift like a God
2. Train like a warrior
3. Sleep like a king

And in addition, you're always either training in Winter Season or Raiding Season.

With these 3 simple rules, combined with Winter Season or Raiding Season, I've managed to totally transform my body. I gained muscle faster than most guys who train at my gym. I lost body fat without ever "dieting" in the traditional sense and I am yet to run on a treadmill.

I can wear clothes that I was never able to before. I look taller because my posture is so much stronger and corrected. I don't suffer from chronic back ache anymore (I had a major back injury in my early 20's). And my sex drive (and opportunities to do something about it) is always through the roof!

Some people that I've introduced Modern Viking to have complained that they don't enjoy the gym and they'll follow the program but they'll substitute weightlifting for squash or soccer.

I'm sorry but that just doesn't work.

Ideally, you wouldn't be in the gym weightlifting - you'd be rowing a boat. Building houses. Hunting for wild game and carrying all 400 lb of it's carcass home. You'd be hauling in fishing nets. You'd be cutting down trees and hauling the lumber back to the saw mill. You'd be drilling swordsmanship and shield wall tactics.

You'd have grown up and know nothing other than the hard and rigorous life of our Viking ancestors.

But modern life has robbed us of most of the opportunities we used to have to build our strong bodies. The best substitute in our modern world is lifting weights at the gym.

Iron man endurance races, rugby/football matches, boxing pad work... these are all very worthy and manly exercises and sports, and feel free to take them up for their other benefits. But if you want a Viking body, you must lift weights. There is no other method as effective for building a lot of muscle mass as quickly on a guy.

I do have specific workout routines (and more available on the book's website at http://liamgooding.com), and there's more information about these in the Lift Like A God chapter. But first it's important to understand these principles, why they work and how to apply them.

As a beginner, you can follow my specific routines and programs, but later you'll also be able to create your own programs to suit your preferences, your lifestyle and what you enjoy.

So many fitness programs or diet plans fail because you're paralyzed when faced with a choice outside of the scheduled and rigid routine. Have you ever tried staying paleo when eating out at a restaurant, or when you download a gym routine but find out your gym doesn't have a smith machine, or you bought the TRX bands but couldn't find anywhere to hang them?

Lift Like A God

Modern Vikings don't follow a *'7 Minute Workout'*, they don't sit in the gym checking their Facebook feed and they definitely don't workout 3 times a week.

You need to remove yourself from the mindset of mere mortals if you want to elevate yourself above them. You need to put yourself amongst the Aesir in Asgard. Would Odin do pushups and sit ups for 7 minutes, 3 times a week? No! He would move mountains, push back the ocean and sweep aside forests - all before lunchtime!

Modern Vikings need to think bigger.

When I started investigating what a Modern Viking training regimen might look like for myself, I researched multiple training methods, the most influential being:

- Bodybuilding
- Strongman
- Olympic & Powerlifting
- Military assault courses
- Boxing & martial arts

One of the biggest surprises I found when I looked at the Gods in these sports compared to regular men was the sheer volume of training they did.

All of the people with that '*Viking Physique*' trained at least 5 days a week, and sometimes 7. They lifted heavy, they lifted often, and they lifted in high volume.

Previously I'd always assumed (and been told by many friends who worked out) that working out in a gym 3 days a week, for 45 minutes, was all you needed to achieve a strong gym body.

Maybe that's okay for mortals and absolute beginners.

But when I did my own research and looked into everyone from Professional Bodybuilders to Army Bootcamp Instructors, they always trained with heavy resistance (i.e., weights) at least 4 days a week. Bodybuilding legend Arnold Schwarzenegger trained 6 days a week for 4 hours at a time! And don't for a second discount that as "Well, he used steroids!". I explore the topic of Anabolic Steroids later (for research purposes - and you can make your own mind up) but you should know that while Arnold did use steroids (as do all professional bodybuilders), the level of steroids available in the 1970's were a fraction of the potency of todays substances. The majority of his gains and recovery were down to great nutrition, solid sleep, and training harder than anyone else.

Olympic swimming legend Michael Phelps trains 6 days a week for 5 hours a day in the water, and also trains weights 3 days a week. And while Phelps might not have the ideal "dry land" Viking physique, the man is undoubtedly a giant and a warrior. Plus as an olympic swimmer, he is definitely not using any steroids or aiding substances. He also eats as much as 12,000 Calories[6] a day!

---

[6] When people say "*calories in food*" they really mean kcal. 1 kilo-calories equals 1,000 calories equals 1 Calorie (with an uppercase C). Don't be confused when reading the nutrition labels on food!

What these guys have in common is that they eat and sleep like a king and train like a warrior. They train as if their life depended on their body's capabilities.

There are thousands of reputable websites and programs that will tell you that training anything more the 3 or 4 times a week is 'over training'. Most of the guys in your gym will lecture you about rest days, muscle groups, and the importance of not "overdoing it".

But with the right diet (i.e., huge and rich in nutrition), the right workouts and the right lifestyle, you can train often and train very high volume workouts. You'll quickly notice your progress overtake that of your gym brothers who warned you about over-training!

Train Like A Warrior

The greatest workout routine is totally wasted if you don't perform it correctly. Just as the simplest workout routine can be insanely effective if you attack it with the right mindset and focus.

To achieve a Viking body, you need to attack your workout as if your very life might one day depend on your gains. You need to recognize that the gym is preparation for a battle-ground, and you need to know that the risk of death is very real if you do not work your ass off.

Kill The Distractions

That means ignoring your phone. Forgetting the music. Ignoring the amazing ass on the girl squatting in front of you. You're in the gym to train for battle - everything else is weakness trying to pull you back into the soft existence that you're trying to rise above.

Circle-Jerking At The Bench

Another example of training like a warrior is how you conduct yourself in the gym. When I first started lifting, I quickly saw the gym as a social place - I would see a group of 4-5 guys standing around a bench press talking and joking and every 5 minutes or so one guy would perform a set. I was the new guy and these guys were veterans, so I'd have to wait for 45minutes or so until they'd finished their circle-jerk[7] and then I could get on the bench and train.

Within 3 months, I was bench pressing heavier than all of these guys, and now when they see me approach the bench, they get out of the way[8].

I get it - your brothers are at the gym and you want to catch up. You want to show off the latest Tinder conquest, you want to talk about last night's football game, you want to get everyone together for a BBQ on the weekend.

But when a Modern Viking goes in to train, they are there to train. Your brothers are extremely important, and building rapport and a bond is critical to a well-rounded Modern Viking. But not on the deadlifting platform, not at the bench, not at the squat rack.

The gym is your battlefield training. An hour spent chatting to your friends will not build muscle. It builds complacency. It cuts into your intensity, into your focus and into time that could be spent making gains.

---

[7] Look this up on Urban Dictionary if you aren't familiar with the term

[8] More precisely, they stand a little back from the bench and watch my full set and discuss how I'm obviously using steroids

Resting Between Skirmishes

You may be thinking, what about during rest periods?

You have just performed your third set on a 570 lb (260 kg) leg press, which is your third out of 8 exercises in today's workout. You have 2 more sets to go. You have 2 minutes to rest.

If your body is capable of wasting oxygen on talking to your buddy for those 2 minutes and you're able to go into your next set and finish it fully, then you weren't lifting heavy enough.

A rest period is not for taking a social break - it's for allowing your muscles to recover from the brutal onslaught you're putting them through before you put them through it again in just a few short minutes. Rest periods are critical - waste them and you risk failing on your upcoming lifts, or having to extend your rests and very quickly ending up with a three hour workout (which is absolutely not possible for 90% of working men!) meaning you'll run out of the gym half way through your workout because you need to pick the children up.

When you walk into the gym, say your hellos. Shake a few hands. Give the nods of respect to your brothers who are turning up and grinding away in their own battles. But then you get to work and you don't look up until the last rep of the last exercise. Reps are work. Rest periods are work. The time walking between equipment is work.

Keep your warrior focus at all times and you'll notice how much easier it is to fit double the amount of work into your routine compared to simple mortals!

Sleep Like A King

"Wake early if you want another man's life or land. No lamb for the lazy wolf. No battle's won in bed."

- The Havamal

It might seem strange that one-third of the Modern Viking workout principles involve lying on your back and sleeping. However, your body actually builds muscle during your sleep. When you sleep, you release Growth Hormone (aka Viking fuel!) and muscle cells repair and multiply.

One of the worst culprits for potential Vikings not making gains is that they simply don't sleep enough for their body to reap the rewards from their workouts. You might do 3 or 4 days of workouts in a row and then go out and get drunk and party with your friends, coming home at 4am. Then you wake up at 8am for work extremely sore, resenting your workouts, not seeing results, and very quickly you start skipping workout sessions because you think that high volume isn't possible.

Lifting like a God and working out like a warrior is only possible if you sleep (and eat) like a king. This important step is how you're able to survive on fewer rest days than weak mortals, it's how you're able to make muscle mass gains faster than mortals, and it's how you'll be able to see cuts and definition without needing to do too much (if any) cardio.

When you start your Modern Viking journey, it might seem somewhat extreme to hit 8 hours of sleep a night - most working professionals sleep for only 5-6 hours with the excuse of *"life is hard, I'm busy, I have children"* (Okay newborn babies suck for sleep[9]) but you need to make a difficult choice on priorities.

Do you want to stay at the bar until 12am with your friend drinking beer 4 nights a week, or do you want to look like a Modern Viking? Do you need to take your laptop to bed at night to watch Netflix, or could you get to sleep 2 hours earlier?

One of the biggest and most instantaneous benefits to your life will come from an increase in sleep - always aim for 8 hours.

Be sure to make up the extra hours with an earlier night rather than a later wake up. Vikings rise early - nets to haul, fields to till, game to be hunted, and enemies to be slain!

You'll recover from the gym quicker and soon the paralyzing aches will be reduced to well-earned soreness. Those few hours in the morning that used to just be coffee-fuelled monotony will now become productive and valuable parts of your day. You'll quickly start to be genuinely exhausted and tired by 10/11pm and happily climb into bed to allow your body to start building your Viking gains.

I personally trained for 5 days a week at the beginning of my Viking journey and took 2 rest days on the weekend. And I deeply needed those 2 rest days! However, once I'd gained a better discipline over my sleep, I was able to increase this to a 6 day training schedule (training each muscle group twice a week) and feel less sore each day too.

---

[9] I haven't created any children of my own yet, but I hear from many people that they exist only to eat, shit and rob you of all sleep

Winter Season & Raiding Season

How you exercise will change based on whether you're currently training in Winter Season or Raiding Season.

By making simple adjustments to your exercise routines, you'll be able to easily switch between gaining muscle and cutting fat, and without any major reprogramming or complications.

Many exercise programs and routines have much more complicated cycles based on *Bulking* and *Cutting*, and there are 1,000 different ways to do cardio and 50 different ways to program your weights.

I just found most of this complexity was at the expense of adherence, and I couldn't imagine Vikings, modern or otherwise, would choose to spend time in front of a spreadsheet that could be spent out in the world living life and getting shit done!

Instead a Modern Viking is always training towards one of two goals: Winter Season or Raiding Season. I'll explain these further, and how they apply, in the following chapter.

Winter Season & Raiding Season

Ancient Vikings were masters at raiding - landing in fast boats and quickly storming unsuspecting villages and towns. They got in quickly, stole everything and killed anyone who tried to stop them, and then tried to get out as quickly as possible.

The fierce brutality in these short raids came from the Viking's long preparation phases back in their home countries in Scandinavia. Vikings would sometimes spend multiple years stockpiling enough weapons, training younger soldiers and building enough boats, before launching a raid.

During Raiding Season, you're rowing a boat a lot. You're fighting a lot. You're probably camping and living on rations or what you can hunt nearby to your camp. You've put in the hard work and preparation and now it's time to reap the plunder and rewards!

Taking inspiration from this cyclical way of life, Winter Season and Raiding Season is an extremely simple but powerful concept I adapted after researching the latest science and techniques in fat loss and muscle building.

Professional bodybuilders have a really intense and complicated system called Bulking and Cutting. During a bulk the general principles are very 'Viking' in nature: Eat lots and lift a lot of weight a lot of times.

However, the complexity surrounding Cutting is insane: during a Cut, a bodybuilder will try to get their body fat below 5% so that they can stand on a stage covered in brown paint, and show off their physique.

Losing body fat becomes an exponentially difficult process. For example, it's much easier to go from 20% b/f to 19% b/f than it is to go from 10% b/f to 9% b/f.

So the complexity, hard work, and science required in bodybuilding is massive. And herein lies the problem - too many guys who just want to look good will try and follow bodybuilding advice, and end up spending more time in forums or medical journals than they will in the gym (or kitchen).

Fitness and exercise is not the end goal of Modern Viking - it's just one of the tools we use to build the lifestyle we want and to add to the sort of man we want to become. If you're anything like me, you don't want to give up such a huge part of your life to live in a spreadsheet that was only designed to work for the top 1% of elite bodybuilding athletes!

So instead of a Bulk+Cut type system, I created the principles of Winter Season and Raiding Season.

Just like with my workout principles to make building your own personal workout routine much easier, I wanted Winter Season and Raiding Season to make it easy and simple to adjust your food and exercise program to meet your goals: either building muscle or building fat.

Muscle Or Fat: Make A Choice

"I turned all my fat into muscle"

"I'd like to lose fat and gain some muscle"

"I don't want to build muscle, just tone it"

People say the most dumb things when it comes to fitness goals. Even trainers in gyms will ask you, "What's your goal?" and allow you to choose something that's biologically not possible.

Here's the scientific truth:

Your body can only be in a catabolic or anabolic state at any one time

- Anabolic: Your body is building muscle mass (and some fat)
- Catabolic: Your body is losing fat (and some muscle)

Unfortunately, your body usually wants to stay in a catabolic state, breaking down muscle and fat into energy. Which means as a Modern Viking, if you want to build any muscle mass, you need to put your body into an anabolic state.

If you don't put your body into an anabolic state, no matter how much you shock your muscles by weight training, they will not grow.

An anabolic state requires both resistance training (i.e., weightlifting) and a calorific surplus. That means you need to be eating more calories than your body is consuming.

Once in an anabolic state, your body can build muscle (plus a bit of fat). The easiest and simplest way to get yourself into this anabolic state as a Modern Viking is to think of Winter Season.

In Winter Season, you're preparing for the cold and harsh weather and test of survival that nature is going to throw at you. You need to eat at every opportunity, because you never know when your next meal will come. Moving around is difficult, breaking ice, climbing through snow, carrying logs to the fire in the great hall - it all requires a lot of work and strength.

Life is hard in winter and now is the time to feed and grow.

However, once the warmer weather arrives, it's time to pull off the furs. That's when you look down and realize that along with the huge back muscles and boulder shoulders, your body thought fit to add a small amount of belly fat over your abs. In fact, it puts a nice insulating layer of fat all over.

But a Viking needs to be fast as well as strong. Fighting in the shield wall requires endurance as well as brute strength. Raiding an enemy requires days of hard work at the oars, and you never know when a hasty retreat might be called. Rushing back to the boat and rowing, quite literally for your life, back down river and onto open waters.

Not to mention the fact that the shield maidens seem to blush when they can make out your ab muscles!

Raiding Season is about leaning up - it's a time to encourage the catabolic state of your body and perform extra cardio work to increase your fitness and endurance. Both for life and for aesthetics.

(The two exceptions to this rule are (1) During your very first few weeks of training, you may notice both muscle gain and fat loss, and (2) When using performance enhancing drugs, it is possible to gain muscle mass without gaining any fat or even losing fat)

How To Adjust Your Workout

Adjusting your workout depending on Winter Season or Raiding Season is extremely simple if you're following my Modern Viking workout routine.

All of your big heavy compound lifts (bench press, squats, deadlifts, lat pull downs , etc.) should look like this:

Winter Season
- 6 exercises per workout

- 5 x 6 reps per exercise
- 3-5 minutes rest between sets

Raiding Season

- 6 exercises per workout
- 5 x 8-12 reps per exercise
- 1 minute rest between sets
- 20 minutes cardio OR add 5 x 10-16 reps drop-sets to each set

Drop Sets or Cardio?

In order to increase the calorific burn of your workouts for Raiding Season, you can either add cardio (rowing, running , etc.) to your workout or you can add a drop-set to each working set.

A drop-set means you complete the regular set, and then without any rest, drop the weight to half and complete another set of 10 to 16 reps.

So if you were doing dumbbell rows, you would take over the 30 kg and 15 kg dumbbell and have them both by your bench. Complete a set of 8-12 reps with each arm, then immediately pick up the 15 kg dumbbell and complete 10 to 16 reps (or to failure) with each arm. That would be one set - rest and then do it another 4 times.

This means you're going to be sweating heavily in your workout and your heart rate will be higher. You should be using lighter weights than you usually use in your Winter Season workouts.

Drop-sets are really just a tool to avoid the monotony of cardio activities, which can become quite boring. Mix it up through the week for variety. Both will achieve the same result - turning a 500-750 Calorie workout into a 1,000 Calorie workout.

How To Adjust Your Diet

Achieving a calorie surplus or deficit can be achieved either by working more or working less, OR eating more or eating less, OR both.

In reality, I find that many guys coming into Modern Viking have always struggled with restrictive diets - those which leave you feeling hungry.

For this reason, I highly recommend not making any huge cuts to your diet and instead making the adjustments in your workouts. I just find it much easier to work harder in a gym than to find the willpower to go to sleep hungry.

Eating For Winter Season

During Winter Season, you should take the policy of "eat as much as you want" to the limit. For example, I ate 5,000 Calories a day during my first Winter Season.

WWE Wrestler and actor superstar, Dwayne "The Rock" Johnson, eats around 5,100 Calories a day[10]. Professional bodybuilders can eat as many as 8,000 - 10,000 Calories a day.

---

[10] http://fivethirtyeight.com/datalab/dwayne-the-rock-johnson-eats-about-821-pounds-of-cod-per-year/

Considering the average guy eats around 2,500 Calories a day, Winter Season is a time to indulge in as much (good quality only) food as you can eat. If its clean and lean, eat as much of it as you want.

You'll gain a lot of mass quickly and you will gain fat too - the trick is to just experiment with yourself and find the 'balance' between how much fat you're comfortable gaining. There comes a point where your body really can't build muscle any faster (around 3 lb of lean muscle per month) so you'll see diminishing returns for unnecessarily consuming extra protein and carbs.

Assuming you're following the Modern Viking workout routine, and you want to gain muscle mass in Winter Season, here's some guideline numbers for a typical 30 year old:

Height	Weight	Calories
5'5"	150 lb	3,700
6'0"	180 lb	4,100
6'5"	210 lb	4,500

Your own specific requirements may be different, and are a factor of age, height, current bodyweight and body composition (percentage fat vs. percentage muscle) and your genetics.

Because of the number of variables that can affect it, that's why I recommend that Modern Vikings start with a baseline figure and just eat.

Your body is pretty damn good at providing you with enough appetite and hunger to fill it up with the right amount of food - Winter Season is just about pushing that appetite and hunger a little bit further (with good food only) and then using a feedback loop every few weeks to make adjustments.

Eating For Raiding Season

Because you'll be making most of your calorific adjustments in your workout, making adjustments for Raiding Season need to only be minor.

You don't need to starve yourself or do anything major - just tweaking down some of the meals ever so slightly is enough to take out the fats. Fats contain twice as many calories as carbs or protein, so only small amounts of them can have a big impact on your daily calorie intake in terms of contributing towards making the calorific deficit.

But seriously, the changes between a Winter Season diet and a Raiding Season diet can be so small, because we're aiming to bring our body fats down from 20-25% to maybe 10-15%. As Modern Vikings who want to look like manly men, we aren't aiming for Fitness magazine body fat levels of 6%!

For example, when I changed my diet from Winter Season to Raiding Season I made TWO CHANGES only:

1. I took the olive oil out of my morning smoothie (2 tablespoons = 250 Calories)
2. I made my 3 daily Whey Shakes with Water instead of Whole Milk (Removing around 600 Calories)

Other than that, I kept eating exactly the same. All the meat, potatoes, vegetables, salads, beans , etc. I wanted. I'm never hungry, but I made a huge calorie deficit with just 2 small changes and then I also followed the workout changes.

Ideal Body-Fat Percentage

Is Raiding Season going to shred body fat at the absolute fastest rate? No. It won't give you the instant "30 day cut" you might have seen on Instagram models pages.

However, for a Modern Viking who has hovered around 18-25% body fat during Winter Season, using Raiding Season to come down to around 10-15% body fat is going to be fun and enjoyable and never once will it feel like an awful diet program or an awful cardio schedule.

At 12% body fat, allowing for variables in genetics, if you've been correctly using weight training on your abs, you will definitely see the definition of your whole abdominals.

They won't have the "shadows" you're used to seeing in Fitness magazines as those guys are usually 6%-8% body fat, photoshopped, and live a full time schedule of dieting and cardio. The only thing in their life is fitness.

At 10-15% b/f you'll definitely notice a cleaner defined jawline, your biceps will carry that *hardness* that most guys want, and the individual muscles across your upper back will be visible. The "boulder shoulder" roundness on your shoulders will be visible. Your thighs will have a subtle definition on your quads and your hamstrings will definitely be noticeably hard and defined.

When you get closer to 10%, you'll notice your lower back looks a lot slimmer and your "love handles" might have disappeared altogether, depending on your age and how long you have been overweight (fat can harden).

Here's the good news: Studies show[11] that most women would choose the physique of a 10-15% body-fat Modern Viking over a 6% body fat fitness model.

And 100% of women would rather date a 10-15% Modern Viking over a calorie-obsessed, cardio obsessed, permanently image conscious fitness model! Girls like a guy who can cuddle up on the sofa with a bucket of KFC every now and then!

Once you've been in Raiding Season long enough to see the sort of body fat levels that make you feel good about yourself and give you the level of cut you like, it's up to you whether you repeat a cycle of Winter Season to add another layer of muscle mass, or if you then stay in Raiding Season, easing up a bit to maintain your current weight and size. Long campaigns can be fruitful!

The key is to find the body size and shape that makes you feel happy, manly and masculine and then stay there (or at least maintain it).

Personally however... I love the idea of seeing how naturally big I can grow. Most of the manly men who I spoke to while researching this book had been lifting (or just living) as Vikings for 5-10 years. Huge physiques take time to build.

Every Winter Season is 10 lb more of muscle. Every year, another layer of muscle, cut the fat, another layer of muscle.

If you started your journey as a fat guy, Raiding Season might take longer as you wait for loose skin to catchup to your muscular physique. If this is you, it's especially important to approach Raiding Season *very slowly*.

---

[11] http://foxhoundstudio.com/blog/fitness-lifestyle/the-ideal-male-physique-%E2%80%94-what-girls-want-want-guys-want-to-be/

Cardio and rapid fat loss are the absolute enemy of fat guys if you don't have a huge amount of new muscle mass underneath to tighten and stretch your skin out.

Make sure you stay in Winter Season, adding huge amounts of muscle mass, for at least 6-9 months, unless you notice your fat levels getting too high.

However if you're a really fat guy, you will actually lose fat during your first Winter Season - because of the adjustment in the quality of your nutrition and the increased metabolism rate from the new muscle mass. But this effect quickly slows down and eventually stops once your body reaches equilibrium, and then you'll be back to choosing to gaining new muscle (at the cost of some fat gains) or burning fat (at the cost of losing small amounts of muscle).

The key is finding the balance and being patient. Your ideal body physique, especially if you're basing it off of fitness professionals or celebrities, will take 5+ years to achieve.

And never try and make all of your progress and gains in one single cycle! A Modern Viking is no good if he's an obese fat fuck, no matter how strong you are. Also be aware that a very high body fat percentage increases your estrogen levels!

And likewise, abs on a skinny guy are just like big boobs on a fat girl - everyone knows it's cheating.

Lift Like A God

Building Muscle Basics

By now I hope you've accepted that being a Modern Viking involves working out. Lifting weights in a gym might be something you already do, in which case a lot of this chapter will seem like stuff you already know.

However, for many people reading this book, you've probably never even been into a gym or if you have, it was to play on the treadmills, maybe you did some strange Personal Training session with TRX bands and a big blue ball, or maybe you just kind of played around on each machine and left after 45 minutes because you felt sweaty.

Or as is very common with a lot of guys coming to Modern Viking - you feel intimidated by the gym and all of the huge bulky Vikings in there. That's totally normal.

Building muscle mass doesn't need to be complicated - it's easy to get it right, but it's also very easy to do it wrong. What's important is you get started today, and you get started correctly.

The 3 requirements to building muscle are:

- Eat a calorie surplus
- Eat enough protein
- Lift heavy weights

The chapters on eating a Viking Diet and Food Supplements will ensure you nail 1 & 2. This chapter is here to make sure you do number 3 properly and don't just waste your time in the gym.

If it wasn't obvious, all three of these have to be happening for you to gain muscle. Simply eating lots of meat, but not working out, will not build muscle. And likewise, busting your ass in the gym, but failing to eat in a calorie surplus, means you won't add any new muscle.

Keeping It Simple

Weightlifting is extremely simple for Modern Vikings. The fitness industry (including personal trainers, home-workout programs and exercise gadgets) would have you believe it's insanely complicated, and you couldn't possibly start training without their help and without buying their gadget.

But Vikings were muscular and strong, and they didn't have the internet. They didn't have excel spreadsheets or smith machines or $10,000 elliptical trainers. They had heavy stuff to pick up and move. They had stuff that needed pulling and pushing. They had life.

The best weightlifting and exercise routine is the simplest one. When it's simple, you are less likely to fuck it up, you're less likely to get tangled up in the complexity and you're more likely to have fun doing it.

By keeping all of the exercises simple and focussing on simple programming, you're far less likely to do anything "wrong" and even more importantly, you're far less likely to get an injury.

I laugh a little inside every time I see brand new guys (who are easy to spot by their $100 Nike running shoes and brand new sports tops) walk into a gym and start trying to train an Olympic Snatch, supersetted with some wild thrashing on the chin-up bar, using elastic bands and lots of twirling to do something resembling a muscle-up, followed by throwing and catching a kettle bell with 3 claps mid-air.

What the actual fuck? Are you trying to kill yourself or what? Stop watching fucked up Youtube workout videos and watch kittens like normal people!

Keeping the moves simple means you'll get them done, you'll need less time to learn the technique and you'll spend more time building muscle. Also, you won't become a 26 year old with the joint health of a 55 year old.

Because I keep my weightlifting routines simple, it means I can play around with them and have some flexibility based on my mood, what I'm feeling like doing, any injuries, or if I feel like working out with a brother that day and adjusting the routine so we can workout together.

I do have a very high-level routine written out to guide my week, and occasionally I'll make adjustments to it, but I don't obsessively record my program and I don't need to carry a diary around in the gym with me.

I'm not saying guys doing that are doing anything hugely wrong, but in my experience, if you can't remember the workout you should be doing today after a quick 2 minute glance at your notebook, then you're spending too much time with your mind in your notebook and not enough time in the gym.

Between 4 to 6 exercises, the same exercises you've done every Tuesday for the last 7 weeks, at the maximum weight you can lift for 5 sets of 6-8 reps each, should not be difficult to remember. It's the same formula every day. The same routine every Tuesday. And so you struggled a bit today on Dips? You don't need to record your feelings, the exact time of failure, your heart rate and how it made you feel in your mood diary. Just move on.

In the spirit of keeping it simple, most Modern Viking workout routines will revolve around 4 very simple primary exercises.

While these exercises are all very simple, they aren't totally retard-proof. I guess if you really are stupid, you could die doing a squat or a heavy benchpress, but then thats Darwinism.

These 4 exercises are the starting point of every program. Everything else you will do will be an extension out from these, filling in some gaps and adding variations.

Safety & Technique

In the spirit of keeping this a book and not an Exercise Manual, there are no diagrams or pictures for the following exercises.

However, please visit the companion website to see diagrams and videos of each of these exercises to help visualize them:

http://liamgooding.com

I also recommend speaking to a fellow gym brother the first time you do these. Ask if you can watch them perform these exercises and if they'll watch you try it. Pretty much every guy is happy to help a new guy out, as long as you have the balls to ask and you show you're willing to put in the work.

The Deadlift

The deadlift is widely regarded as the single best exercises for adding the most amount of muscle mass.

A deadlift is just picking up something really heavy, and then putting it back down. Imagine picking up a log, or picking up a boat, or picking up a rock.

It's an extremely "functional" exercise in the sense that learning to deadlift is learning how to pick something up - it translates into real life and the real world.

It's performed by loading up a barbell with the big weight plates (45 lb or 20 kg plates). You'll quickly find that you can lift a lot of weight with a deadlift - your first target should be to lift your bodyweight (6 - 12 months of training) safely and for reps. Your 3 year goal should be to deadlift 2 x your bodyweight safely and for reps.

A deadlift works all of your leg muscles, your back muscles, your arms, shoulders and your abs. In fact, there's barely a muscle in your body that isn't worked by a deadlift.

Because of this, you get huge amounts of HGH (Human Growth Hormone) and Testosterone release when you perform this exercise - your body basically panics and thinks *"Fuck we need to grow bigger and stronger - fast!"*.

This is why it's a great mass builder - it stimulates your whole body to grow.

Completing a deadlift safely isn't difficult but it extremely important... because the risks are lifelong lower back injury.

For safety reasons, I really can't stress enough how important it is to work through these exercises with someone experienced or at the very least, watch lots of video guides first!

Make sure to stick your ass out and arch your lower back - think Silverback Gorilla! When you pick up the weight, the first part of the movement is lifting with your legs, and then you finish by driving your hips forward (squeezing in your glutes) and pulling your shoulders back to finish in a strong "I just fucking did this!" pose.

Of course your upper back muscles, and to a lesser extent your lower back muscles, are engaged in a deadlift. But they should not lead the core work - that's how you fuck it up.

Common mistakes guys make are that they try and lift too much weight, which causes them to bend over in their back (curling their back like a cat stretching). This is almost guaranteed to cause a serious injury - it only takes one rep.

When you become more experienced at deadlifts, you can start to use a weightlifting belt to help you with your form and to help get more work done.

Vikings would actually wear a wide leather belt almost identical in function to a lifting belt, and for the same purpose. Sometimes when you're tired and the thing you're lifting is heavy, you can forget to fully arch your back gorilla-style. The belt just helps with this by maybe 20%, saving you from fatigue and possibly from an injury.

However, never rely on a lifting belt.

Deadlifts should be performed heavy but safely. This means driving up slowly, but if you can't lift the weight in 2-3 seconds, you're probably using too much weight and at risk of your back losing good form. (Assuming you aren't testing a 1 rep max).

Also many injuries happen after the lift, when you're putting the weight back down. Many gyms and trainers will tell you to slowly lower the weight, however this isn't because they give a shit about your back. It's because they want their equipment and floor to last longer and their miserable members to not complain about "noise".

(If you ever see anyone complain in your gym about noise: banging, grunting, screaming , etc., please punch them in their dick and tell them to quit. They don't belong here)

A deadlift works you out the most when you lift it up. When you lower the weight, you're still performing work but you're also putting yourself at bigger injury risk.

Allow the weight to drop in a controlled manner but don't let the weight pull you down - if you feel even the slightest twinge, just drop it. I recommend using weights called Bumper Plates (speak to the guys in your gym) which are designed to be dropped safely. Or, put a few folded yoga/stretching mats under the plates. Or join a new gym.

The Benchpress

Infamous as the "Bro" exercise of choice. Guys of all types, Viking or not, feel the urge to have a big chest. And for good reason - both men and women disproportionally judge the muscularity of a man (and by connection, his status and value) by the size of his chest.

It also plays a serious role in all of your functional movements as a man and as a Modern Viking. A fully developed chest works with your back and shoulders to create a solid posture. It allows you to move the heaviest furniture in your house. It allows you to push back in the shield wall.

Most of the way you will have seen a benchpress performed is on a purpose-designed benchpress, with a frame to hold the barbell while you load the weights. A spotter will help you to lift the bar off the frame, and maybe help you with the last 1-2 reps and to get the bar back on the frame.

However, for nearly all new Modern Vikings, I recommend you do not use the barbell benchpress (at least for now).

Instead, use a regular flat bench and use dumbbells to perform the bench press exercise instead.

Doing a dumbbell benchpress has a few advantages:

- You can usually get started with a much smaller weight, and then watch your almost weekly progress as you use progressively heavier dumbbells each week

- You do not need a spotter - if you find yourself about to fail on a set, you can just throw the dumbbells to the side with no risk

- Most gyms have dumbbells that are 5 kg to 40 kg. This means you can progress from a 10 kg to a 80 kg benchpress, which is good for at least your first 2 years

- Because of balancing the weights and the range of motion, training with dumbbells will correct any small weakness and imbalances you have as a weightlifting beginner

- It allows you to slowly build in confidence in the gym - the benchpress can feel like an intimidating piece of equipment for many beginners

- You can still go heavy with the dumbbells by using a spotter who can help you get the last few reps out of your sets

Once you're comfortable and making strong progress with dumbbell bench press (and all of it's variations) you can start working with heavier weights on the barbell (always with a spotter).

Injury risk from dumbbell benchpress is very rare, because there's very little to fuck up! On the barbell bench press, the main risk is failing and getting "trapped" under the bar. Because if this, you should always do 2 things:

1. Never lift heavy without a spotter
2. Never use collars on the bar. In an emergency, you can tilt the bar and allow weights to slide off

The two variations from flat bench are an incline bench press (so you're kinda sitting up, with the bench at a 45° angle) and a decline bench (where you're laying backwards on a sit-up type bench with your feet anchored). These variations help to make sure you build those big "panel pecs" as they help to build and define the very upper and very lower part of the pectorals.

The Back Squat

The third, and perhaps most hated big lift you will be doing is the squat. A squat works all of your lower body (calves, quads, glutes) as well as your abs.

It involves squatting down as if you're taking a dump behind a bush, but you also have a tree log balanced across your shoulders.

To perform weighted squats, you'll need to use a Squat Rack, Power Cage or Smith Machine in your gym. However you can also buy pretty affordable squat stands if you're doing your Modern Viking workouts at home.

Squats, like deadlifts, have a potential for injury if not done correctly. Also, anyone who has had a previous back injury (like myself) will never be able to train this exercise to their full potential.

However, it is not a difficult exercise to perform. And just like with deadlifts, the key is to leave your ego outside and start with a very light weight and slowly progress over months and years to using a heavier weight.

The key things to remember about performing back squats is to make sure you go lower in the squat (even if it means using a lighter weight) as the very bottom of the squat is where your glutes will be engaged, and building a strong and balanced lower body is key to achieving the rounded Modern Viking physique.

Keep your feet around shoulder width apart, with your toes pointing forwards, and come down in a slow and controlled squatting movement. It might help to think more as if you're trying to sit on a bench behind you rather than sitting on a stool between your legs. Rest the barbell just behind your shoulders (not on the base of your neck) and get used to supporting it in position rather that letting it press down into your spine.

As you come down, remember everything about the deadlift - gorilla back! Stick your ass out and arch your lower back with your chest up. Don't allow yourself to bend over forwards - if you are, that means the weight is too heavy.

Once you get comfortable with the squat, the main variations you'll want to add are a front squat (or a goblet squat) and a leg press (if you have a machine in your gym).

Goblet squats involve holding a heavy dumbbell in front of your chest while doing a squat. Or very similar, you can support a barbell in front of your chest. These just shift the location of the weight, and take some of the pressure off of your spine.

Leg presses mean you change your whole body position so that you're pressing a weight up at an angle while sitting back into a chair. Leg press machines come in lots of different designs, but generally speaking they move more work to the quads and calves rather than the glutes. However, they have much less chance of lower back injury and usually have safety catches in case you fail a rep.

The Pull Up

The fourth main exercise for a Modern Viking is extremely intimidating for most guys, and even after training for a long time, it can remain a challenge.

Pulling yourself up on a bar (with a wide, overhand grip) is a huge workout on all of your upper back and arms, but particularly for your lats. Your lats are the primary muscle that gives you that huge "V" taper. Biologically speaking, that V-taper is what women are programmed to look for in a guy and there's no quicker way to achieve a Viking look - whether you're a fat guy or a skinny guy - than working on that shape.

It's also just an extremely important part of your strength - if you can't pull yourself up and over the side of the boat, you're going to get left behind in the water during hasty retreats!

The problem with training pull ups is that there is a huge learning curve - most guys just coming into Modern Viking, big or skinny, will struggle with pull ups. You may not be able to do 1, never mind 10. I honestly couldn't do a single pull up when I started and even now, they're one of the hardest exercises I do!

However, the trick to building up to training pull ups is to use these 3 progression exercises, training each of them at least 2 days a week:

1. Jump up and then hold yourself at the "top" of the pull. Hold yourself here for 5 seconds, and then drop

2. Jump up, and then slowly lower yourself, trying your best to make the lowering move last for at least 3 seconds

3. Jump up but try and use your arms to pull in the move too. Just fall back down and repeat immediately again

I see heavy guys in the gym, ripped in muscles and looking like big strong Vikings, who still struggle to perform a set of 10 pull ups. It's an exercise that will always test your back strength against your current bodyweight, so don't be put off with the slow and hard progress.

As well as the progressions above, you can also perform chin ups (i.e. with an underhand grip) which will be a bit easier because they allow you to use more of the strength in your arms. Also, most gyms have an "assist" machine, where you can kneel on a plate and add 10 kg to 70 kg of assistance. This means you can perform the same natural pull up move, but with only a part of your bodyweight. Also, training with a Wide Lat Pull Down machine allows you to achieve a similar effect.

Pull ups have zero risk of injury and most guys intuitively figure out good form. Grab the bar, pull yourself up.

Compound Vs. Isolation

Each of the 4 core exercises I just explained (Deadlift, Benchpress, Squat and Pull Up) are examples of compound exercises.

This means that performing them works multiple muscles - they're big exercises that require a lot of work to complete one rep.

This is great for Modern Vikings who want to achieve a lot of real-world strength. You (probably) aren't training to stand on a bodybuilding stage looking like a strange biology accident - instead your goals are to get big, get strong and look like a manly man.

Compound exercises are great for this because they maximize the testosterone and Human Growth Hormone release in each lift. They're also extremely tiring, meaning they use a lot of calories to perform - which is great for maximizing the "work done" within a fixed 1hr gym session.

However, in-between your compound lifts, there are small muscles that contribute to your strength and physique and also smaller exercises that can help to improve your performance in those big lifts (called accessory exercises).

While the core of your program should always be built around big compound exercises, and definitely as a beginner you should focus 80% of your time and energy on these exercises, eventually you will want to start "filling in the gaps".

For example, almost each of the 4 big exercises contribute to your bicep development. They all tax your biceps and make them work to some degree. But eventually, you'll want to add some focussed bicep work to really grow some guns!

Bicep curls, hammer curls and concentration curls are examples of performing slight variations on bicep curls that are good for training your biceps to failure at the end of a workout. These moves don't require a lot of 'work' in the sense that your biceps are relatively small muscles and you're usually moving quite a small weight (10-20kg) through a small distance. So isolation work won't release testosterone, growth hormone or burn enough calories for significant fat loss.

Each gym session should start with the big compound exercises, and then complete the smaller isolation exercises towards the end of the session. This means you save your maximum energy for the bigger moves and then can focus on really "emptying the tank" towards the end of the workout.

However, don't worry too much about isolation exercises in your early stages - so much of your growth and progress will come from big compound movements and their variations.

Sets And Reps

The best method for lifting weights for optimal muscle growth is to work in Sets and Reps.

A rep is performing one complete movement of the exercise. A set is a series of reps, performed without rest. Then you take a rest after one complete set (usually 30 seconds to 5 minutes, depending on the routine) and then perform the next set.

There are many different systems and opinion on the best combination of reps and sets.

Should you perform 3 sets of 10 reps (30 reps total) or 5 sets of 6 reps (30 reps total)? It's the same total amount of work, so it shouldn't be any different, right?

Well, it isn't quite that simple.

Shorter sets allow you to focus on fast-twitch muscle cells. These are your strongest muscle cells, but they tire much quicker. In contrast, slow-twitch muscle cells aren't as strong, and don't grow anywhere near as much as fast-twitch, but they can work for much longer.

Also, lactic acid accumulates in your cells as they work. This builds up very quickly under extreme workload (like a weightlifting set) and your body usually needs a few minutes to recover. So completing a set of 6 reps versus a set of 20 reps would mean you'd really feel the burn towards the end of the set. That burn is your muscles getting drenched in lactic acid and struggling to get enough energy into them so they can perform correctly.

With that simple bit of science out of the way, what does a Modern Viking need to know?

For maximum muscle growth, you always want to be working with heavy weights and high volume. So for Modern Viking workouts, you will pretty much always work an exercise for 5 sets of 6 reps for any compound exercises, and 5 sets of 8 reps for simpler isolation exercises. This is a good "all round" system.

During Raiding season, you might add 2-4 reps to these numbers and lower the weight - but during Raiding Season you aren't trying to build muscle, you're trying to *maintain* muscle while working in a calorie deficit.

You might see guys in your gym working in very long sets - 15 reps or more. Assuming these guys aren't idiots and they know what they're doing, then they are most likely trying to maximize their lean cut - i.e.. burning as much fat as possible. Or they are bodybuilders who are 3+ years into their journey and are following a maximum-hypertrophy bodybuilding program.

5 sets of 6 reps is a balanced amount of work for an exercise to build both strength and mass. Using the heaviest weight possible, it allows you to get a huge Viking pump in your exercises, and flush your body with testosterone and growth hormone.

If you're ever doing a warm up set (lift with a light weight to stretch through the range of motion of the exercise) or you're completing bodyweight exercises for cardio (or Viking Bootcamp) then you will use higher reps per set. Again, that's because at these times your goal is not to build muscle but usually fat loss, flexibility and mobility.

Failing

If you start a set and you feel like you're going to fail on rep 4, immediately drop the weight by one plate (or one increment) and finish that set. Then put the weight back to the original for the next set, complete as many as possible, then drop the weight again. Never allow yourself to just "quit" and drop a weight if you can perform at least half of the set with the weight.

Likewise, if you get to rep 6 and you don't feel exhausted, you probably need to move the weight up. You need to choose a weight so that reps 4,5 and 6 of your 4th set are a real struggle. And reps 3,4,5 and 6 on your final set are almost a total failure. That's how much these 5 sets should exhaust you.

Resting Between Sets

When you're working 5 sets of 6 reps, your rest between each set should be around 3 minutes, and as long as 5 minutes if you're training squats or deadlifts. This will allow you to go for maximum strength and performance in each set. Don't think that you're doing yourself a favour by resting for shorter - you'll only be training with an inferior weight (and therefore work the muscles less) if you take shorter rests.

When you're in Raiding Season, shorter rest periods are OK to keep your heart rate a little higher during the workout. But remember that you'll be performing slightly longer sets but with a lighter weight.

Viking Basic Bootcamp

While I endorse an intensive training week for Vikings, with those 4 big exercises at the foundation, I realise that everyone will be coming to their Viking Body transformation from different places.

Some guys may already be weightlifters, some may have never stepped foot in a gym before, some guys may play a lot of sport and do other activities.

Whatever your situation, I suggest completing a simple Viking Bootcamp first for 4 weeks before you worry about the full Modern Viking muscle building routine.

This will allow you to work out all the simple movements and identify any obvious weakness areas, and also just get you more slowly used to the gym.

During the Bootcamp you'll perform a full body workout every day you train, which is different from a normal Modern Viking routine where you give the major muscle groups a chance to rest before working them again.

However in a Bootcamp, your goal is to train to *be able to train*. That is, you want to get your fitness, flexibility, movement and habits in the right place before you start worrying about following the bigger weightlifting routines.

Each of the exercises are like an introduction to the exercises you'll be doing in your regular workouts.

For convenience, a PDF of Viking Bootcamp is available for download on the website http://liamgooding.com

Viking Bootcamp is only 4 days a week, and around 30 minutes each day. It doesn't matter how you spread these 4 days out over you week, just get used to the idea of prioritizing time for the gym.

A note to advanced guys - if you look at this and think *"I can easily do that, I'm way beyond that!"* then that's awesome. All I ask is you just run through the 4 days of workouts, condensed into 2 days, to confirm that there are no problem areas in your flexibility or mobility.

You should go and do this in your gym - even though it requires minimal equipment, you want to start getting used to the routine and habit of going to the gym, meeting guys there, getting used to fitting the gym into your life , etc.

Day 1

1. Jumping pull ups: 5 x 8 reps
2. Jump and hold pull ups: 5 x AMRAP
3. Air squats: 5 x 8 reps
4. Pushups: 5 x AMRAP
5. Mountain climbers: 5 x 12 reps
6. bench dips: 5 x 8 reps

Day 2:

1. Jumping chin ups: 5 x 8 reps
2. Jump and lower pull ups: 5 x AMRAP
3. Lunges: 5 x 8 reps (each side)
4. Wide pushups: 5 x AMRAP

5. Plank hold: 5 x 15-30 seconds

6. Smith/Table rows: 5 x AMRAP

Day 3:

1. Jumping pull ups: 5 x 8 reps

2. Jump and hold pull ups: 5 x AMRAP

3. Air squats: 5 x 8 reps

4. Mountain climbers: 5 x 12 reps

5. Pushups: 5 x AMRAP

Day 4:

1. Pull ups: AMRAP

2. Jumping chin ups: 5 x AMRAP

3. Lunges: 5 x 8 reps (each side)

4. Narrow pushups: 5 x AMRAP

5. Plank hold: 5 x 15-30 second hold

6. Smith/Table rows: 5 x AMRAP

AMRAP = As Many Reps As Possible

For the pushups, if you can't do 1-4 reps in the set, then put your knees on the floor (but lean forwards). Ideally you want to be able to complete 4 - 8 reps per set.

For Smith machine or table rows, lay under a smith machine bar (or under your dining room table if it's strong enough, or under a barbell in the squat rack) and pull your body up. You can try experimenting with different angles of your body to change the difficulty. The point is to pull (or row) your body up until your chest touches the bar. These can be killer at first, so don't expect to do many reps.

Building Your Routine

Once you're ready to start following a full weightlifting routine, its important to think about your goals as a Modern Viking.

You aren't training to stand on a bodybuilding stage and you're not training to be on the cover of a fitness magazine. However, you do want to achieve the following:

- A wide and thick back
- Thick and rounded shoulders
- Wide arms (biceps and triceps)
- Thick and balanced quads and glutes
- Wide and thick chest
- Strong abs
- Low enough body fat that your muscles are discernible and you're healthy

To build big and strong muscles, you're going to need to work them hard but also give them enough time to rest.

Remember, sleep like a king!

I'll go on the assumption that you are willing to commit to your Modern Viking transformation and dedicate 6 days a week to your transformation.

A 6 day training program for maximum muscle gain would look like the following:

- Day 1: Back & Chest
- Day 2: Shoulders & Arms
- Day 3: Legs & Abs
- Day 4: Back & Chest

- Day 5: Shoulders & Arms
- Day 6: Legs & Abs
- Day 7: Rest

To make this 6 day program work and to avoid injuries or overtraining, the exercises are varied between the different days.

For example, one day the chest exercises might be focussed around using a flat bench, and the other day using decline & incline benches to hit the chest muscles from a different angle.

This would be an ideal and very intense Modern Viking program, requiring a lot of calories, but yielding awesome results.

With a bit of adaption, it's easy to see how this is actually just a week in the life of a Viking:

- Day 1: Rowing, hauling nets, shield wall drills
- Day 2: Picking stuff up, building a house, axe drills
- Day 3: Carrying things, hauling back a deer carcass, wrestling
- Day 4: More rowing, more fishing, more shield wall drills
- Day 5: Axe drills, sword drills, throwing spears
- Day 6: Carrying grain sacks, framework
- Day 7: Drink with the boys, spend time with the wife

I recommend this 6 day program for most Modern Vikings who want to achieve maximum results in size and muscle mass. It really does build the Viking physique most men are looking for, and will definitely put your body on the right track to building the body most women are looking for[12].

---

[12] Women's ideal male physique is different from the physique most men want for themselves. It's a cruel trick of biology

If you look on my Instagram account (@modern.viking) this is the exact program I have been following for my own workouts, with the exception of the first few weeks I did a general Viking Bootcamp of full body workouts every day that I could.

For specific exercise routines and workouts, please visit the website. I didn't want to clutter this book with too many tables and diagrams.

The Mind-Muscle Connection

One of the best practical tactics to gain focus during your workouts is performing each rep with your mind connected only to that specific muscle group you are using. Everything else is noise.

Every major professional bodybuilder, including Arnold Schwarzenegger, praises the value and effectiveness on what's called the "Mind-muscle connection". This means trying to mentally focus on contracting a very specific muscle so that you can be laser focussed about which muscle is performing the work, and therefore which muscle will become exhausted (and therefor grow).

I'll be honest - it sounded like a lot of whispy-washy nonsense when I first heard about this technique!

But when you perform an exercise like a high Lat Pull Down, you soon notice what it means. On this exercise, if you simply grab the bar and pull it down, you're subconsciously engaging every and any muscle that can help with the movement. Biceps, triceps, shoulders, lats. At the apex of the movement (the maximum contraction) it's far too easy to only be working the lats about 60% of their maximum capacity. However, if you perform the rep again slowly and try to mentally picture your lats contracting and pulling on your arms to pull down the bar, and try to mentally black out every other muscle group in the chain, at the apex of the movement you feel a hard and dense contraction in the lats.

Once you start doing this you'll realize how much concentration it requires. Everything else will soon fade away into the background. It's like gym meditation, but without the chanting.

This mind-muscle connection took me around 3 months before I started to feel it in certain lifts. But within weeks of working out with this absolute focus, I noticed the difference in my pump, in the hardness of those muscles, and the boost it added to my overall workout focus.

Choosing A Viking-Friendly Gym

As you know by now, most compound exercises (the best type) to simulate a Viking exercise lifestyle only involve a few simple things: barbells, dumbbells, pull up bar, bench & benchpress.

I still don't know what most exercise machines work - some of the gyms I've been in look more like a NASA innovation lab than a gym.

At the end of the day, it's about going in and picking stuff up, pulling stuff around and pushing stuff.

The Right Equipment

Too many people judge a gym by how many treadmills and ellipticals they have. Do you realize, a typical commercial treadmill costs $30,000, whereas an Olympic Barbell and Bumper plates costs $2,000?

So when you see all of those treadmills in your gym - guess how they're paying for that? Yup, with your overpriced membership and by cramming as many members in as possible.

When your gym has simpler equipment, it means as a business they can afford to offer a cheaper membership and can afford to focus on having members who want to make serious changes in their body. These are the sort of brothers you want around you while you're training!

An ideal gym for a Modern Viking has at least a few bench press stations, a smith machine (a good multi-use backup for if the place is busy), at least one squat rack (or power cage), and a few olympic sized barbells, with plenty of 45 lb (20 kg) weight plates to go around.

The only good piece of cardio equipment that is essential is a high quality rower. This is the staple of every Modern Viking's cardio come Raiding Season!

Ideally the floor should have a strong rubber matting - the sort of matting where you know they are casual about weights being dropped and thrown around.

The Right Attitude

The best time to checkout a potential gym is 6.30pm to 9pm. These are the peak hours and will give you a good feel for the sort of people in there and the sort of attitude everyone has.

Things to look for:

- Do guys seem comfortable dropping dumbbells and making noise?
- Do guys seem to feel comfortable about grunting or screaming the last rep or two out?
- How many people are just loitering around on the weights floor versus actually getting shit done?
- Do you notice many people saying "hi" to each other? Or are most people just keeping to themselves?

It seems strange to look for these things (and maybe it seems strange that I've included them in this book!) but I was amazed at the difference it made to my workout, my progress and my attitude towards the gym when I switched gyms. Feeling comfortable and feeling like I could really train 'like a Viking' had a massive difference, especially in making sure I gave my all for 2 hours a day, 6 days a week. I wanted the gym to be where I went to battle, and battle is messy and noisy and sweaty and it's not alway pretty!

The Modern Viking Diet

"Shun not the mead, but drink in measure."

- The Havamal

How Vikings Ate

Vikings were mostly farmers and fishermen. But their homelands are a harsh place, with unforgiving terrain and extreme climates. The yield from farms would have been very low, so we know that simply getting enough nutrition would have been hard.

This was one of the main driving factors for Vikings choosing to settle in the much richer and fertile lands of England and Ireland, where growing and fishing enough food was much easier.

With most of their protein coming from fish and farmed animals, Viking men would need to have been extremely resourceful when it came to getting enough calories. For example, a favourite Viking breakfast was pig fat mixed in with porridge oats!

Cold weather, lots of manual labour, and also trying to build the body of a strong and muscular warrior would have been difficult. Vikings needed to consume a ton of protein and calories from fats and carbohydrates. While also working extremely demanding schedules. In summary, life was hard!

While there is nothing particularly exciting or appealing about a Viking diet, when compared with fun and exotic diets such as Mexican food, Chinese food or Indian food, there is a wonderful utility and efficiency to eating like a Viking as a man.

Thinking about food in terms of what you need rather than what you want. Focussing on food for the fuel of life, the fuel of growth and the fuel of battle.

But also, knowing when to fill your long hall with all of your brothers and having a feast to make even the Gods jealous!

The Problem With Most Existing Diets

When I started to work on my Modern Viking transformation and what my diet should look like, I started my exploring most of the existing fixed diets out there. Vegan, Raw Diet, Atkins Diet, Paleo Diet, Gluten Free Diet, Juicing Diets… there's so much bullshit out there, it was a crazy minefield!

I started to dive into everything from a research perspective. As a 28 year old guy, I'd already been independently controlling my own groceries and food for 10 years, I'd followed intensive training schedules before as a Kickboxer training 7 days a week, and I'd also watched my body become fat, skinny, and everything in-between.

I was already quite familiar with the problems and incompatibilities that many diets had:

- They were expensive to follow
- They were inconvenient because they required too much planning and preparation each week
- They were antisocial because of how limiting they were when eating with friends
- They did not handle big appetites well
- They did not promote naturally high testosterone levels
- They had too many strict rules and caused a lot of anxiety if you "fall off the wagon"
- They were wrapped up in too much marketing to really dig into the science and proven benefits or were backed by a for-profit company that just made everything a bit suspicious

I knew that these reasons had always caused me to mess up with diets before. While I was fully aware that any successful Viking Body was going to be achieved 50% in the gym and 50% in the kitchen, I was a long way from anything perfect or ideal if I simply followed an existing diet out there.

So I started to build the Modern Viking Diet, borrowing things that worked and throwing out things that didn't. I experimented and made notes and made sure the eat element was "battle tested" with my crazy lifestyle, work schedule and requirements. I also knew that if other guys were going to be able to follow the diet, it needed to be able to adapt to your lifestyle and your personal preferences, so I didn't want to be too specific and too rigid.

Instead of coming up with fixed meals, fixed ingredients and fixed programs, I created the Modern Viking Diet as a series of principles and guidelines. Each one designed to make it easy to build the Modern Viking Diet into your lifestyle, while still making sure that you're benefitting from the thousands of hours of research I'd already done and saving you from the thousands of blog posts and scientific studies I'd read to put this together.

1. Eat as much as you want
2. Food is fuel
3. Feast with friends
4. Eat Stuff with faces
5. Eat Vegetables

Following these simple principles, which I'll explain in more detail later, will mean you'll be getting all of the benefits from the leading science in the nutrition industry. You'll also be getting a diet that can fit with even the busiest of lifestyles. It's been built specifically for men to maximize testosterone levels naturally. You'll never feel hungry or like you need to "cheat" on your diet.

This diet will stop feeling like a diet at all - it'll just be the way you eat as a Modern Viking.

Eat As Much As You Want

The first principle to a Modern viking diet is probably the most shocking, but also the most exciting, of them all. Seriously, eat as much food as you want.

If you follow all of the principles of this diet, and you're following a Modern Viking transformation properly, then you really are going to need a hell of a lot of food.

Whether you're a huge obese guy, or a tiny skinny guy, this rule is the same. I really mean it, eat as much food as you want. Now before you stop reading and think that I'm a crazy lunatic who's trying to turn you into a fat fuck, let me explain why this is the number one and potentially most important principle of the Modern Viking diet.

Speak to any bodybuilder, strongman or professional athlete, and ask them what they eat. They will begin to list off a huge list of food, probably eating a meal every 2-3 hours. Rice and chicken breast, broccoli and steamed fish. Whey protein shakes with oats. These guys know that for their bodies to go through their gruelling training schedules and grow muscle (or maintain their muscle) they need a lot of calories and a lot of protein.

Protein for the muscle. Calories for the energy and recovery.

When you start working out like a Modern Viking, your body is going to get shocked into growth mode. This growth requires huge amounts of protein - much more than you're probably eating right now.

If you're a really fat guy, you've probably being eating a lot of calorie dense foods (sugary and fatty) such as cakes, donuts, fried meats and fast food. You weren't doing any physical exercise so all of these calories were just getting stored as fat. Now that you're working out, whether for Winter Season (focussing on adding muscle) or Raiding Season (focussing on losing body fat), you're going to be tearing up your muscles which requires huge amounts of protein (either to build the muscle or to maintain it). This means eating a lot of rich protein sources - way more than your previous diet used to contain.

The second issue if you're a really fat guy, or like me just a very tall guy, is you probably have a huge appetite. You're literally used to eating lots of food. So the best way to ensure you're going to stick to the Viking Diet and enjoy it is if you can keep eating as much food as you want, and eat whenever you're hungry.

Once you're following all of the Modern Viking Diet principles and all of the Modern Viking program, you'll realize that you really can't fuck it up, no matter how much food you eat, because the food you're eating is all great food that your body can utilize!

And now consider the other extreme scenario - you're a really skinny guy who's always struggled to put on weight, *"no matter how much I eat!"*. This is usually for 2 reasons: your genetics have gifted you with an extremely fast metabolism, so your body just burns through it's calories faster, or (and most common) you just think you eat a load but when you actually analyze your calorific intake compared to your lifestyle, it's just not enough.

You can't gain muscle (i.e., gaining weight) unless you eat a calorific surplus. This means after your day is done, your body has burned through the calories it needs just to live, and you've done your exercise in the gym, you've walked the 2 miles to work, and you've done your days work, and you've had sex with your wife , etc., you still need to make sure you consumed at least 300-750 calories more.

So in order to transform into a Viking, you need to get used to eating a lot more food. You need to train your mind and your body to have a bigger appetite. So you need to eat lots, and in some cases, eat even if you don't feel hungry. Most professional bodybuilders or professional strongman competitors, who are probably the most extreme cases of trying to gain muscle, talk about the struggle of having to eat when they aren't hungry. They just have to push beyond what their body *thinks* it needs, and keep on eating!

You aren't a professional bodybuilder, but if you're an extremely skinny guy, you may need to do this for a few months until your body gets used to eating 3,000 Calories a day.

You might be wondering about the risks - will eating as much as you want mean you're going to just get fat?

No, because the principle is eat as much as you want, not eat as much as you want *of whatever you want*.

Of course, there are some foods that you just need to stop eating - they just aren't part of what you need as a Viking. I'll explain more about this later, but accept that you aren't going to be eating a 12 box of donuts. But once your refrigerator is full of all of the foods a Viking eats, sure go nuts. Eat everything.

The sort of food that a Viking eats is nutritious, provides constant energy levels throughout the day and prevents any energy spikes, full of all the protein you need to gain muscle and recover quickly, and most importantly, it's all extremely satiating. That means it makes you feel full.

This means you'll never be battling hunger with your Viking diet, so you're unlikely to ever break it. Hunger on any diet sucks. Hunger is a powerful urge for most people that we just aren't used to feeling in a Western society. When we feel hungry, we quickly change into a Scarcity Mindset, where all we can think about is getting food.

Food Is Fuel

The second principle of the Viking diet is probably going to be as unpopular as the first principle is popular. *Food is Fuel* means you need to learn to change your attitude and emotional connection to food. This is probably the most difficult, but most important, principle to the Viking diet.

It's an extremely challenging mindset to master, and I think after 7 months of practicing this, I'm about 75% of the way there.

Changing the way you see food, from something that brings enjoyment and emotional pleasure to something that simply brings nutrition, means you'll be able to start connecting with food simply as the building blocks you need to grow, to workout, or to fight. You'll stop seeing the colorful marketing of the billion dollar food industry and you'll start seeing protein, carbs and fats. You'll see a 1 hour workout. You'll see a 4 hour hike.

Because that's all food is - it's a means to an end (when we look at it without emotion). It's fuel for our engine. You don't care about the marketing messaging. You don't care about how pretty it looks. And you don't care about spending a long time putting it in your stomach.

You just want to get good quality fuel into your body.

When you drive your car to the gas station, you're putting in gas/petrol so that it can drive for another 500 miles. You don't put in the purple strawberry flavored gas, you don't put in the gas from the strange sketchy looking gas station, and you don't put in the gas endorsed by Beyonce. No one likes long lines at the gas station either - filling up with gas is a simple act of utility.

You just want to get good quality gas into your car engine.

As you start to see food in this way, you'll realize how liberating it can be and how much better your relationship with food will become. You'll stop stressing about cooking. You'll get your groceries done much quicker. You'll save money on overpriced luxury foods. You'll buy much better quality food (in terms of nutritional value).

The sugary crap that made you fat will naturally disappear. The hassle of preparing a healthy meal for an hour will soon disappear when you realize that you can just eat the stuff in 10 minutes.

Food is Fuel is a simple principle but it actually has a few different meanings in the Modern Viking Diet:

- *Food is Fuel* means you shouldn't worry about each meal being a "proper" meal that comes together beautifully on a plate

- *Food is Fuel* means you should look at food at its macronutrient level: how many grams of protein, fat and carbs are in this? And what are the total calories of this?

- *Food is Fuel* means you should stop wasting time eating food and just get it in your body and get on with your day

- *Food is Fuel* means you should care about the quality of the food that goes into your body

- *Food is Fuel* means you should stop using food as a personal reward

Transitioning to this mentality does take time. Emotional triggers with food, particularly comfort food, have been built up in your body over years and years, and overwriting those will take time.

However painful, it is an absolutely essential component to the Modern Viking Diet, and in my experience it has been the most defining characteristic of changing from *diet* to *lifestyle*.

I discuss in the supplements chapter how *Food is Fuel* helped me to wrap my head around protein & Meal Replacement shakes, which now make up for 25-50% of my macro-nutrient requirements on busy days (i.e., days where "life" doesn't allow time for food-meals).

This attitude to food is also one of the most essential principles in diets of almost every professional athlete/bodybuilder/actor I researched.

Food is fuel means you appreciate that food is a utility and eating that food is only providing your body with stuff that it needs. However... this leads me onto the next principle which may seem like it totally contradicts everything I've just said...

Feasting Is Social

"Always rise to an early meal, but eat your fill before a feast. If you're hungry you have no time to talk at the table."

- The Havamal

Vikings knew how to have a good time, and one of the most famous parts of Viking culture is their love of feasting. Local Viking government was based around the idea of a Jarl (a Lord) who ruled the village/town from his large hall. While the people on his land served him, to an extent, he also served them in that one of his duties was to host regular feasts in his hall. Feast would be held for any special occasion or traditional celebration.

Feasting allowed the village to unwind, to sort out grievances and feuds safely, for games and entertainment, for flirting and fun. They were an essential part of the village functioning properly and flourishing.

A true Modern Viking needs to have feasting in his life! Feasting is the one time when eating food is not about putting fuel and macronutrients into your body. The food (and ale) is merely the lubricant for the social interaction. It's just an excuse to get together!

Food is Fuel - when you're eating breakfast, lunch, snacks… you're just putting the fuel into your body and getting on with your day. And for 75-95% of the times you eat during your week, this applies.

But that one time on a Friday evening when you eat out with the guys from work. Or on the Sunday lunchtime when you go over to your parents house and all of your family gathers around the table for a big dinner together. Those times are not about fuel - they're about coming together.

And those times shouldn't be made more difficult by the diet you've chosen to follow.

Yes, it would be great if everyone in your family and all of your friends ate like a Viking, but this is not the time to tell them that. If you eat at a restaurant that only serves Burgers or Tacos, don't irritate the whole group by arguing with the waiter for 10 minutes about why he can't create a separate meal that doesn't come with fries or bread and adds double meat. Order the best food you can get that fits your fuel requirements for that meal but honestly, don't stress about it. Focus on why you're there - the social interaction.

For the really hardcore out there, you may be thinking that this means you're not being "strict" on your diet and you'll make slower progress. That one meal which caused you to take in 900 Calories where you'd only planned out 750 Calories, or where you couldn't get enough protein because the meat portions on all of the dishes were really small.

Here's the logic though - in the grand scheme of the 28 to 42 meals a week you eat (depending on if you're eating 4-6 meals a day), that 1 meal in the week really isn't going to matter. As a working guy (or in college) the chances are that you don't eat with friends or in a big social group that often. Once or twice a week, at most with friends.

A Modern Viking Diet is about eating to become a Viking, not eating to become a professional fitness model. It's much healthier overall and promotes a balanced state of happiness for you. Use those times at Feasts to socialize with your friends, to ease tensions with your irritating brother, to get drunk and swap stories about past conquests of the female nature.

Most people have been out to dinner with that one friend - the vegan, or the Raw diet guy, or the paleo guy. The guy who just creates a fuss and just generally pisses everyone off by trying to preach his bullshit diet onto the rest of the group for the next 25 minutes.

People don't go out to eat with their friends to get lectured about the food they're eating. If you're friends want to be Modern Vikings, they can buy this book (another coffee for me!) and choose to follow the Viking diet. But when they're out in the bar, they might just want to eat a greasy burger with a mountain of fried onion rings and a double ice-cream milkshake washed down by a few shots of whiskey. And you should feel free to do the same.

Enjoy your feasts, because the slightly more relaxed nutritional choices you'll make really aren't going to damage your overall progress that week, but they will provide you with amazing experiences with the people who are important in your life.

The caveat to this principle - if for some crazy reason, you find yourself eating out with friends a lot more than a few times a week, then you may need to pull back a little. However in my experience, an ambitious guy who is working on something in his life doesn't feast that often. Grabbing lunch with a friend isn't a feast. Eating an evening meal every day with your wife at home isn't a feast. During those times, stick to Food is Fuel - you've just got company along for the ride.

Stuff That Had Faces

Getting Your Protein

If you're going to build the body of a Modern Viking, you're going to need to eat a lot of high quality protein. While you can find some protein in many foods, there are more easier to find and higher quality protein sources than eating other animals. Cows, pigs, Tuna, Birds, Squirrels, Snakes… No matter what, if it had a face, then it's high in protein.

A vegetarian is going to find it hard to become a Modern Viking, and a vegan is going to find it almost impossible.

It's possible to get protein from plant sources - the most popular being Soy, Rice or Pea protein. Each of these are made by removing most of the carbohydrates until a very concentrated protein is left behind. While these protein sources will do the trick, you'll need to consume a lot more of them because the protein is lower quality (your body can't utilize all of it properly). But most importantly, no Viking ever woke up and said *"Hey you know what, I really want to devour a juicy piece of concentrated, powdered Soybean!"*.

Unfortunately, in todays modern society of billion dollar food industries and heavily industrialized meat production with extremely questionable practices (I'm looking at you America) eating stuff with faces isn't as simple as it should be. Non-organically farmed meat is pumped with antibiotics (which among other bad things, will increase your estrogen levels) and other bullshit chemicals, and thats before we dive into the profit-driven practices that drive most meat supply chains. Unfortunately the topic of sourcing meat and fish in modern society is bigger than this book alone, but a few simple rules that will help:

1. Always buy organic. The price is higher but you can afford to buy less meat

2. Organic chicken & turkey is better value for money than beef

Raising Testosterone

Studies have shown that eating meat (and eggs) increase testosterone levels in men. Testosterone is vital for any Modern Viking (I deep dive into the subject of testosterone in a separate chapter) but in particular for significantly increasing muscle growth and fat loss.

In one particular study, researchers had 2 groups of men follow a 12 week weightlifting program. One group ate meat whereas the other did not. At the end of the 12 weeks, only the meat eaters had shown significant muscle growth and fat loss. (The meat eaters were also probably much more fun at a BBQ).

While there are many things you change about your diet to naturally increase testosterone levels, eating meat is probably the most critical.

Eating Stuff That Came From Stuff With Faces

A small extension to this principle, is to eat stuff that came from stuff with faces. This means eggs, milk, yoghurt and probably the most critical - whey (I cover whey isolate protein more in the Supplements chapter).

Not only do eggs increase testosterone, but all of these products are extremely affordable and extremely convenient protein sources. While most cheese is too high in fat to eat much of (and if you're being offered cheese out in a restaurant, you should almost definitely turn it down) other dairy products are amazing fuel for a Modern Viking.

Yoghurt, particularly natural yoghurt from skimmed milk (with no added sugar) is an extremely low calorie, high protein and delicious dessert. Just use common sense and avoid the high sugar, high fat desserts. Yoghurt contains slow-digesting protein so it's a great snack to eat in the evening before bed, so your body can slowly release the protein through the night.

Eggs are incredibly convenient - in todays world you can safely eat raw eggs without salmonella (I've been eating raw eggs every day for years) but even if you're worried about this, you can scramble eggs within a few minutes or buy pasteurized egg whites (I usually keep a bottle or two of egg whites in the fridge and pour 2-4 egg whites into my whey protein shakes - you can't tell they're in there.)

With the exception of cheese, all of these products are very budget friendly and particularly good for college students who are struggling to make their protein requirements and can't afford to buy much organic meat in their groceries. Whey isolate protein, eggs and egg whites, and skimmed milk are all extremely cheap per 1 g of protein.

Eat Vegetables

The two key ingredients in a Modern Viking diet are stuff that had faces, and vegetables. It really is as simple as that.

But I said vegetables, not *fruits* and vegetables.

While this principle should be common sense, unfortunately misguided health advice lately means that many people think they should be eating lots of "fruit and vegetables". They encourage their children to drink fruit juice and think they're being healthy by making themselves a fruit smoothie for breakfast.

Just because fruits and vegetables both come from plants, does not mean they're both good for you.

Fruit is nature's dirty little secret. All brightly colored and tasting absolutely delicious. So fucking delicious…

It's also cheap as hell in the supermarkets and available in a thousand different ways… Smoothies, cakes, yoghurts, ice cream. Billion dollar food companies make billions of dollars because they're clever as hell. They've slowly conditioned you into thinking fruit is good for you - after all it comes from nature and contains vitamins! So then when they put fruit into their high sugar, high fat ice cream, you think its healthy. When they sell you a 'Nature's Awesome Fruit Smoothie', you think it's healthy and good for you. *"Look, it has anti-oxidants and vitamins!"* You totally miss the fact that you're consuming 750 Calories of pure sugar (fructose), without any protein.

Vegetables on the other hand also contains vitamins and minerals, but they're lower in sugar. They're high in fibre which means your body can properly handle fat digestion (and you know, you can take a regular dump). Vegetables help to make you feel full. They provide slow release carbohydrates. They block estrogen production in men (Modern Vikings should become good friends with broccoli for this benefit!).

Vegetables are never going to win the Most Delicious Competition against fruit. But a Modern Viking should aim to eat a big portion of vegetables with every meal. Yes, every single meal.

The next time you eat a salad, you should be aiming to eat about a large mixing bowl just of vegetables (mixed spinach, lettuce leaves, cucumber, red onion , etc.) Without ruining it with a ton of dressing, a hungry Modern Viking can consume this huge bowl of vegetables (with a chicken breast on the side) and feel completely full and satiated but you'll have consumed less calories than just a few pieces of fruit. You'll also have taken in an entire chemistry lesson's worth of vitamins, minerals and beneficial awesomeness.

In fact, I am yet to come across a vegetable that isn't awesome for you, or a vegetable that you aren't able to consume huge volumes of (great for big guys in Raiding Season).

Diet Willpower

Many diets are an "all or nothing" mentality. If you're following Paleo, you need to eat Paleo 100% of the time and anything else is "cheating" or "falling off the wagon". People on a Gluten Free Diet kick up a huge fuss in Starbucks when none of the sandwiches on offer are on gluten-free Rye bread, and they can only shop in overpriced whole foods stores.

This absolutist mentality is, in my opinion, one of the main causes for anxiety and stress in diets and the reason for creating the cheat day or cheat meal.

When you're on a diet so strict and so absolute that you need to give yourself a cheat meal, in my opinion you're living on a temporary diet. Not a sustainable lifestyle change.

When I created the principles for the Viking diet I was determined to put together a diet that didn't need cheat meals. I didn't want to feel stressed or anxious if I ever slipped away from the rulebook. I didn't want to be the guy who causes the whole group to change restaurant because this one didn't fit my ridiculous diet.

Making a big lifestyle change like Modern Viking is hard. It requires a lot of willpower and there are going to be plenty of opportunities for you to doubt yourself and have set backs.

You don't need any more, especially ones caused by failing your diet because you finally got fed up of asking if they have gluten free bread available for the 1,000[th] time.

I believe that the small sacrifices you make by being less strict with the rules of Modern Viking have huge payoffs in terms of giving you the best chance possible to stay adherent to the transformation overall.

Would you rather be militant strict on a diet for 3 months, and then go back to your regular lifestyle, or would you rather stay 95% strict on the Modern Viking Diet and stay on it for years? Occasionally giving yourself a break, like when Feasting, or when you're feeling low energy so you eat some fruit, or you're really hungry and the only thing nearby is a McDonalds.

Modern Vikings don't care whether they eat 4 times a day or 6 times a day. If your job doesn't allow you to take multiple breaks, no problem. Have one epic feast in your lunch break. If you really can't stand fish, no problem. Stick to chicken and beef and take a fish oil supplement. If you really just can't stomach most vegetables, just invest in a NutriBullet and blend a bunch of vegetables with a banana and drink your vegetables.

Dieting Technology

For the most part, following these principles will just work without any meal plans, logging calories or looking up foods. Eat as much meat and vegetables through the day as you want and you're almost guaranteed to be eating enough protein for a good number of calories. Adjust your training based on whether you're in Winter Season or Raiding Season and you'll gain muscle or lose fat based on how you're training.

For your first 6 - 12 months as Modern Viking, this works fine.

However, after your progress begins to slow down, you need to start being a little more accurate with your calorie intake. Specifically, when you're gaining muscle you want to aim for 500-750 Calories extra each day (after considering your exercise on that day) and when losing fat you want to aim for a 250-500 Calorie deficit that day.

It's perfectly possible to do this by creating a pre-defined meal plan for the week in a spreadsheet on even just in a notebook, and spending some time with a calculator and ingredients labels to add up the calories of each meal. However, a much easier way to do this is to log your food (and therefore add up the calories) using an app called MyFitnessPal (free for iPhone and Android).

This app allows you to log all of the food that you eat (it has a barcode database of most supermarket food) and then adds up the macronutrients and calories that you consume through the day. This means it will tell you how many 'calories you have left today' and how many more grams of protein you need to eat today to meet your target.

While I genuinely don't think it's essential for a Modern Viking to track calories as accurately and strictly as a professional bodybuilder or fitness model, I would say this app was useful in getting a feel for nutrition.

After a while, you just start to get a *feel* for 200 g of protein and 4,000 Calories spread over 5 meals looks like. You start to learn portion sizes and macronutrient profiles of the foods you eat most often.

Sure, just from forgetting to add the latte you had at lunch or by rounding errors, you might be 100-200 Calories away from the exact calorific deficit/surplus you were aiming for, but I don't think most guys who are lifting hard in the gym are going to see this affect their progress.

Personally, I found living by the exact numbers every meal-time of every day a little bit stressful. Again, back to my point about the stress and anxiety caused by the "all or nothing" of diet regimens. Macronutrient tracking in MFP is something I usually use for a few days to check that I'm still 'on track' and then I'll leave it for a week or so. If I decided I wanted to get below 10% body fat, or I wanted to train for a 300 kg deadlift, then I'm sure I could use the app to get the absolute maximum efficiency out of my diet.

But being a Modern Viking is about a well rounded lifestyle and sometimes sacrificing that last 5% in work can make the whole process much more sustainable and enjoyable.

Diet Supplements

Cutting Through The Bullshit

This chapter could be a controversial topic with a lot of people who bought this book - I know it certainly divided the room during all of my research interviews.

The problem is, supplements just don't feel very Viking. There's something not very traditional or pure about using supplements for some people.

But I never wrote this book on how to become a Viking. It's about how to become a Modern Viking. And just how as a Modern Viking I used the internet to research almost everything, I used my smartphone to track my macronutrients and calories, so too as a Modern Viking do I rely on food supplements to maximize my training and/or compensate for my busy lifestyle.

The fitness and food supplement industry is huge - and I can honestly tell you that the vast majority of it is inflated and based on selling snake oil. Seriously, the majority of supplements available in Sports and health supplement stores will not have any noticeable benefits for 99% of the people who take them.

Sure, each bottle and each product and unique combination is "Scientifically proven to maybe help...".

I have a background in Astrophysics, so I'm more familiar than most when it comes to experimental process and scientific research papers. This came in extremely useful when I started digging into the research and science behind the supplement industry for my research for this book!

There is simply so much bullshit out there, with commercially sponsored studies working with tiny groups of participants and then using ambitious language to present the findings. The companies backing the studies know full well that once secondary and tertiary publications pick up the results, "Vitamin X may be linked to muscle cells" quickly becomes "Take Vitamin X and you will gain muscle quicker!" and suddenly Vitamin X supplements are everywhere for $39.99 a bottle.

And then there is the situation where a supplement actually might increase performance/results but only in the most extreme of cases, i.e., top level athletes who need to get that extra 3% of performance. In sports and fitness, increased performance becomes exponentially harder the more you improve. For example, losing your first 5% body fat is much easier than the next 5% (or even 1%). This creates a group of people who will endorse the benefits and results of Vitamin X - but then the average Joe on the street thinks they also need to go out and buy it.

Modern Viking is about an entire lifestyle transformation - it's not purely a fitness program and it's not about becoming the top 1% of Professional Bodybuilders or Crossfit Competitor.

Over-supplementing isn't going to cause any negative health effects - it's just extremely expensive! It's far too easy to spend $500 per month on supplements, when everything after the first $50 is a total waste.

The following are supplements that have both a lot of extremely conclusive research behind them, and I have also anecdotally used them for a considerable amount of time (including cycling on and off to confirm) and would stand behind them for Modern Vikings.

I've discussed the supplements in terms of the priority order I think you should use them. For example, if you only have a spare $30 a month, I suggest you spend it on Whey Isolate before you worry about Fish Oil or ZMA/ZMB.

Natural Supplements

Each of the following is a food supplement that I would consider natural - and by that I mean each of them can be found by eating regular food. However, it's just that either the quantities or price of eating the real food is prohibitive, or, just simply inconvenient.

Whey

Whey Isolate is a by-product of cheese production (it comes from Cows Milk). This stuff is almost entirely protein, and extremely high quality protein (high quality means it is both easily digestible by your body and most of it is utilized - much more than other protein sources).

It's sold as a powder (usually flavored like Strawberry or Chocolate) and you just mix it with skimmed milk or water. Mixing it with milk usually tastes amazing and will be indistinguishable from a regular milkshake. Mixing it with water means you don't need to think about the extra sugar and fat in the milk (ideal for Raiding Season) but it usually requires a strong Food Is Fuel mentality - drinking chocolatey water just isn't great.

However, after a month or two of drinking Whey with water, you soon forget about it.

Why is Whey so awesome and in my opinion, practically essential for most Modern Vikings? It comes down to price and convenience.

A tub of the best quality zero-sugar & zero carb (my recommendation) Whey Isolate will cost around $65. This will provide 30 x 40 g servings of top quality protein. This is roughly the same price as getting the same amount of protein from cooked chicken breast. So you aren't wasting money on "overpriced protein".

Couple this with the simple convenience of making a Whey protein shake up in 2 minutes versus cooking 2 chicken breasts, and whey isolate quickly becomes one of your best friends in terms of getting enough high quality protein as a Modern Viking.

You have to eat your protein every day (2 g of protein for each 1 kg of your bodyweight). For me this means eating at least 200 g of protein each day. Most days I don't track so accurately, so I like to eat a little over when it comes to protein. I'm pretty good at eating things with faces for every meal, but sometimes I'm busy or the day has just got away from me. It's not unusual for me (and many guys) to have days where I miss some meals and I might only eat 2 proper meals in the day.

On these days, I know I can smash 2 or 3 Whey protein shakes, taking up 2 minutes each, and get 80 g to 120 g of extra high quality protein.

Also, as I've sunk further into my *Food Is Fuel* mindset, I find myself using Whey Isolate (with oat flour) to account for at least 50% of my daily protein intake. I just don't care that much about eating food when I have so many other amazing and exciting things to do in my day!

There are a few things I've learned about Whey protein that's worth mentioning:

Always buy the best quality protein you can. The cheaper Whey Concentrate proteins are less refined and contain lots of extra crap - almost all of these that I tried gave me an upset stomach. Also the math usually didn't make the product any cheaper - when you read the label and discover only 70% of the product is actually usable protein, saving 20% on the price of the higher quality protein doesn't actually ad up!

Rotate flavors. Supplement companies are great at coming up with so many different delicious flavors, and one of the best way to ensure you don't get fed up of your whey is to rotate your flavors. I keep multiple tubs of whey at once so that through the month I'm actually having 4 or 5 different flavors.

Don't buy any kind of "All In One" supplements or "Mass Gainers". These are usually just Whey Protein mixed with some kind of added carb and always work out much more expensive than eating regular food or just mixing in your own carbs (see oat flour next).

When you mix your shakes in specially designed shaker cups that come with your protein (or sold in storeS) make sure you immediately rinse out the shaker afterwards. If you buy your protein from a local store where the owner can get to know you, you'll usually get a new shaker cup for free with each new tub - this isn't by accident. It's because after around a month, the plastic cups start to stink no matter how many times they go through the dishwasher!

I just need to emphasize - you do not need to use whey protein. This section is about supplements - they supplement your diet. However, you need to get your protein and while I would love it if you could eat stuff that had faces for 4-6 meals a day, it's not always easy with the demands of modern life. I find that investing in whey protein saves me tons of hours in eating and cooking time each month, and I can use that time to do way more interesting things like pillaging and plundering new countries!

One side note - some people struggle with digesting Whey Isolate protein. While it should be your first choice, assuming you've tried a few of the best quality brands and still have trouble with gas or an upset stomach, you can now purchase other great powdered protein such as Beef Isolate, Casein or even vegan options like Soy Isolate and Pea Protein. These vegan options are inferior (in terms of protein digestibility and usability by your body) to Whey Isolate, and there are some studies (though not conclusive) presenting some issues around using these protein sources.

Oat Flour

The next "supplement" I absolutely recommend isn't really a supplement in that it's just a really simple food (oats) ground to a flour to make it easy as hell to eat. Oats (aka porridge, oatmeal) are extremely Viking - if you want to get extremely traditional in your Modern Viking transformation then I really do recommend Bacon with Porridge each morning for breakfast!

However as a Modern viking, particularly during Winter Season when I eat around 5,000 Calories a day, I quickly became reliant on Oat Flour to meet my food goals for the day while still getting on with my life.

There are three amazing things about oat flour, and it's the reason why it's the most popular ingredient in "Mass Gainer" products (along with Whey protein):

It contains very high quality, low GI carbohydrates. this means your body gets a slow and constant release of energy when you use Oat Flour to get yours carbs

It contains protein and very high quality protein too (the protein in Oats is actually around the same quality as protein in fish!). 100 g of Oat Flour available in supplement stores contains around 18 g of protein!

It mixes in water/milk along with your Whey Isolate and can be drank instantly. You don't need to cook it like you do rice, pasta or potatoes. This means you can just smash it down in 2 minutes

Oat flour is extremely affordable - around $8 per 1 kg in most food supplement stores. The reason I don't recommend buying any Mass Gainers as a Modern Viking is that you can simply buy your own top quality Whey Isolate and your own Oat Flour and combine them yourself, saving around 75% on the price of commercial Mass Gainers!

As with getting your protein from Whey Isolate, you don't need to use Oat Flour at all. If you can eat rice or sweet potatoes through your day with your meats, then I recommend it! But once you try using Oat flour for a week and you realize how much more convenient it is, while still eating a natural and nutrient-dense carb source, you just get used to it.

Sure, it's another step towards Food Is Fuel, but Vikings have shit to do. Would you rather spend your day chopping up sweet potatoes, or would you rather smash down a Whey+Oats shake and then go out and get on with pillaging?

One note - you can buy separately flavored oat flours. I don't recommend using Oat flour without whey, which is always flavored, so I really don't see the purpose in these more expensive flavored oat flours. You also need to think about the added sugar and artificial flavorings added to these. I'd stay away - these, along with the huge array of overcomplicated "Mass Gainers" are just one example of the supplement industry trying to make a very simple product seem more complicated so that they can extract more gold coins from you.

Creatine

Creatine is a supplement that scares away some people because they just don't really understand it fully. Which is ironic considering it's possibly the most researched and studied sports supplement out there!

It's the most researched because it works - supplementing creatine makes you stronger. That's a fact. If you can lift a particular weight for 10 reps, with creatine you'll be able to lift it for 12 reps.

Hundreds of studies have proven this, and I've anecdotally tested it myself (I cycled off of creatine for 1 month and saw all of my lifts decrease by around 15-20%).

But what is creatine?

Creatine is an amino acid that allows your muscles to get more energy when they need it the most. It's produced naturally by your body, just not in very high amounts. It's utilized by your muscles during explosive lifts and towards the end of your sets, when you otherwise would be too exhausted to lift any more. It allows you to squeeze out an extra few reps (or the same set with an extra few kg in weight).

Being able to work harder for longer means you can train your muscles just a bit more, and therefore make gains a bit faster.

This means you don't need to supplement Creatine - you can gain muscle and get stronger by going to the gym and following your Modern Viking workout routine without it. It's just that creatine will help you squeeze out a bit more - it'll give you the edge on the battlefield that could mean the difference between loss and victory.

If a Viking lord was offered a chance to make his húskarlar[13] 20% stronger, do you think he'd take it?

You *could* avoid purchasing a creatine supplement if you ate a lot of organic, grass-fed beef. I recommend supplementing with 5g of creatine a day - to get this amount of creatine from food, it would require eating 1 kg of grass-fed steak each day. Not ideal on your wallet or diet!

Creatine monohydrate is extremely cheap - a $10 tub will last you a couple of months. You just mix a teaspoon in a glass of water each day - that's it.

Some pre-workout supplements (see the chapter on Viking Juice) contain added creatine, so this is something to watch out for. Taking more than 5 g of creatine shows diminishing returns, so you could be wasting money if you're taking Creatine on days where you use pre-workout.

My problem is that I don't usually know if I'm going to use pre-workout until about 5 minutes before I head to the gym (sometimes I just don't feel like I need it and I try to avoid pre-workout unless I really need it) whereas I take creatine *every* morning. So I specifically buy a pre-workout that doesn't contain added creatine (basically just caffeine).

When you start to take creatine, you will quickly gain 1-2kg in weight. This happens because creatine causes your muscle cells to hold a little more water, so the weight you'll gain at first is just added water. After that initial weight gain, any weight you gain on creatine is going to be muscle (assuming you workout).

---

[13] The Old Norse term for house troops

You do not need to cycle off of creatine for any health reasons - you can safely continue to take creatine indefinitely. However, if you do cycle off of it you will notice your strength falls away by around 15%. I tested this myself (also just to anecdotally confirm the strength boost) and I saw this happen within a week of stopping my creatine intake. As soon as I went back on Creatine, within a week my lifts were back to the same levels as before and I've been on it since.

The most common criticism for creatine when I started researching it was kidney damage - however I couldn't find any reputable piece of published science to support this. All of the concerns around creatine causing kidney damage seem to be anecdotal discussions on forums (along with muscle cramps and stomach cramps) but I couldn't find any studies supporting these.

Paul Greenhaff, Phd. Professor of muscle metabolism at the University of Nottingham, UK, **has been studying the effects of creatine for over 20 years.**

"If there were any major adverse side effects of creatine, we would have seen them by now".

If anyone ever tells you creatine can be dangerous, please ask them to link you to published research to support it.

Fish Oil

As a supplement, fish oil is something that you really should try and get from your diet naturally. Eating fish is awesome - it's full of protein, Omega 3 and tastes delicious. It's also extremely Viking of you to eat plenty of fish - Vikings were fisherman after all!

However, some people just don't like fish or don't eat it regularly enough. If you aren't eating fish at least 3 times a week, but you're training weightlifting, then you should purchase a fish oil supplement. It's not expensive and it takes a few seconds to take a few caps of fish oil each morning.

Why is it so important?

Besides the multiple health benefits of fish oil with studies suggesting an improvement in neurological health, kidney and liver health, we're primarily concerned about the health of your joints.

Weightlifting can be stressful on your joints, and not just for older guys. Even at 28, after just 3 months of weight lifting I'd started to experience soreness in my wrists, elbows and shoulders. After researching joint health and realising I wasn't eating enough fish, I started to use a fish oil supplement and within 2 weeks the soreness in my joints had mostly gone. Nothing about my training changed (I always followed correct warm up and stretching routines).

The only thing I changed was the fish oil supplement.

There is a huge market behind fish oil which means there are a lot of overpriced branded products on the shelves. From what I found in research, there is little difference between the different products so purchasing a simple fish oil supplement is fine (around $10 for a month).

Many younger guys might not feel like they need to supplement with fish oil, and that's fine. If you've never felt joint soreness it can be difficult to justify that extra expense each month. Or if you just tend to eat fish a few times a week, you'll be getting enough from your food.

But my advice for any guys who start to feel a bit of soreness, or who don't mind dropping an extra few bucks a month, would be to add fish oil to your supplement stack.

Viking Juice

This is a pretty controversial chapter, however in the spirit of education I wanted to include it because I know it came up in my research a lot (and too many people interested in this book have assumed that all guys who look like Vikings *"are just injecting steroids"*).

I had my own questions about anabolic steroids - I'm open to anything that brings us closer to the Aesir. As a guy looking to become a Viking and not a competitive olympic athlete, I was open to finding out what they were, how they worked, and why over half of the famous fitness personalities on Instagram were using them.

If you have no intention of using pro-hormones to unnaturally boost your testosterone levels or growth potential, I still recommend you read this chapter so that you are properly educated about them. Life is so much more depressing when we are ignorant to things that just because they *"aren't for us"*.

Just as I don't believe in magical spells and wizards, it doesn't mean I shouldn't learn about Christianity and other religions.

I haven't used steroids (referred to in fitness communities as *"staying Natty"*) and I don't think I will. However if there was something out there that could make me stronger, smarter, faster, better... basically worthy of a seat in Asgard, then I'd explore it and consider the risk-vs-rewards.

I also moved the information about Pre-Workout supplements into here. Pre-workout isn't a pro-hormone anabolic steroid **at all**, however it does provide an "almost inhuman" performance boost but at the cost of potential side-effects. It's also a slightly tongue-in-cheek joke, as once you get further into the fitness lifestyle you start to hear more jokes and banter about *"the guy who took 3 scoops!"*

For this reason, I felt like it should be categorized as Viking Juice. Something which an ancient Viking almost definitely would use, but something that a Modern Viking should only use with your eyes open to the full story.

Pre-Workout Supplements

Pre-workout is amazing. It's like having 3 cans of Red Bull injected into your eye balls by a Shark riding a flying flaming Lion, while heavy metal music plays in the background.

Depending on the brand you buy, it's usually some concoction of Caffeine, Creatine, Beta-alanine and straight up voodoo.

OK but seriously you should check each ingredient in your pre-workout labels as some of them will just make your face-numb and your balls tingle, but provide no benefit to your workout. Some pre-workouts are amazing, others are simply an excuse to put strange chemicals into a tub of asthma-inducing powder cloud and sell it to chumps for $40.

When I first started my journey in becoming a Modern Viking and I discovered a good Pre-Workout, it felt like the most authentically Viking Berserker thing I could use without doing something illegal. Take this drink, feel invincible for the next 2 hours, and worry about the damage to your kidneys and heart later.

The primary problem with pre-workout is that they rely on your Kidney and Liver to deal with the chemicals in them. You're taking extremely concentrated doses of stimulants, amino acids, vitamins and minerals. People can suffer from cramps, headaches, vomiting, itchiness and irritability, problem sleeping, high blood pressure, chest cramps, and of course the most serious, kidney damage.

In case there's any doubt about whether you're taking a natural product or something made in a lab, pre-workout is usually neon green or bright blue. It's pretty much what I imagine the Incredible Hulk's ejaculate to look like.

Because pre-workout is amazingly effective at getting the mental boost you need to get your ass in the gym, it will start to lose its effect over time (chemically speaking - your body builds a tolerance to it) and also psychologically - you don't want to build a Mindset of thinking you can't workout unless you've taken pre-workout.

For this reason, I recommend trying to only use pre-workout on days when you really need it. For me, this is usually 1-3 times a week out of 6 workouts. Some bad weeks I might use it every day, some weeks where I'm just on a natural high I won't use it at all.

One thing to be aware of is that many pre-workout supplements contain creatine, which you're probably already buying and supplementing. Creatine monohydrate isn't expensive, so you can usually save quite a bit of money by buying a cheaper pre-workout that doesn't contain creatine and just add your own. Hitting 5 g if creatine a day isn't difficult so there's really little need to have it in your pre-workout too.

Pre-Workout isn't illegal. It isn't an anabolic steroid. But it does make you feel like a Berserker!

Anabolic Steroids (Pro-Hormones)

Anabolic steroids (aka pro-hormones, gear, juice) are pharmaceuticals that increase your bodies testosterone levels and human growth hormone levels (HGH) to enable you to build muscle faster than your body's natural limits.

In most countries, taking anabolic steroids without a prescription is illegal. However, because some people are offered anabolic steroids and Testosterone Replacement Therapy by their doctor, and may be curious as to how taking these treatments may affect their Modern Viking transformation, I wanted to run over some basics.

Obviously I'm not a doctor, and I don't use these steroids myself. But it's going to be impossible to enter the world of weightlifting without coming across steroids eventually and particularly as Vikings who are always looking for an edge to become stronger than your enemy, I thought you should at least be primed with the basics.

Injecting Vs. Oral

First things, steroids come in two forms: oral or injectables. The stereotype of people taking steroids is sticking a needle in their ass, but you can also get oral steroids where you simply swallow a few pills.

I think being able to sidestep the requirement of inject is a big reason for steroids growing in popularity, however this is not good!

Oral steroids, like anything you ingest, are handled by your liver. And all oral steroids are extremely hepatotoxic (toxic to the liver). Oxandrolone/Anavar is the least hepatotoxic but still bad. What this means is that your liver is absolutely smashed by taking these drugs and as an older man, you are more likely to develop liver cancer or liver disease.

When prescribed by a doctor in the low doses that they were intended, the hepatotoxicity is manageable. But when bodybuilders take them at 5-10x the recommended dosage, the hepatotoxicity is very high and you can do some serious long term damage.

I came across a lot of bodybuilding forums where "newbies" to steroids were discussing taking a series of oral steroids, and the unanimous advice from seasoned steroid users was always to not bother. If you really do decide, after all of the warnings and side effects and risks, that you want to take steroids, then **do not use oral steroids**.

No matter how appealing the convenience may be, the damage to your liver is very real and very serious and unavoidable.

If you are too scared of a small needle then you really do not deserve to get bigger.

Testosterone/TRT

With the idea of using oral steroids out of the way, that leaves most guys considering injecting Testosterone (usually in the form of Testosterone-Enanthate or Testosterone-Cypionate).

Some men may also have been approached by their doctor for (legal) Testosterone replacement Therapy (TRT). This is becoming an increasingly common treatment in the US and Europe. Each week, you get a Testosterone E injection from your doctor which gives your body a big boost in testosterone. It's prescribed for older guys, however the market for testosterone that you can inject yourself, at home, in larger quantities, is booming.

Almost every bodybuilding forum I used to research steroids contained links to small independent pharmaceutical labs who produced injectable Test-E to purchase via mail order.

The benefits of injecting testosterone are huge: you will gain muscle mass much quicker than your bodies natural limit. You'll feel stronger in the gym. Your body will burn fat faster.

However, the rewards come at a cost.

You need to remember that you are putting a hormone into your body artificially. The problem is that this affects your bodies natural hormone balance, and after a while it stops making its own testosterone (referred to as *being shut down*)

This means that once you stop injecting testosterone, your testosterone levels will plummet. And if you've been on an extremely long (or indefinite) cycle of Test-E injections, this shut down is permanent. You natural levels may never rise again and you will need to continue to pay for TRT for the rest of your life.

In less extreme cases if you only injecting the testosterone for a 10 week cycle, your natural testosterone production will return within 4-12 weeks of stopping. However, you will need to use anti-estrogen medication like Tamoxifen (brand name Nolvadex) and Clomiphene (brand name Clomid) to prevent the crazy hormone imbalances from producing huge estrogen levels and causing feminine bodily side effects such as gynecomastia (breast tissue growing under the nipple).

When your natural Testosterone levels return, they will not be at the extreme high levels they were at while injecting, so the muscle mass and strength you gained will eventually disappear as your body's natural hormone levels just cannot sustain it. Keeping a lot of muscle mass requires a lot of testosterone, and your body will fall back to a balanced equilibrium.

The basic lesson here guys, is once you start injecting testosterone for muscle and strength purposes, you're pretty much making a life-long commitment, both biologically and financially.

Dianabol, Winstrol, Deca, HGH , etc.

The most common anabolic steroids that you will come across are Dianabol, Deca-Durabolin and Winstrol. These are pharmaceutical steroids that aid in muscle gain and are usually taken in combination with injecting Testosterone-E. They are extremely popular in bodybuilding because they are extremely cheap - for just a few hundred dollars you can purchase a cycle (a course of treatment) of these steroids.

All of these steroids have **serious negative side effects** and using any of them is a very delicate process that requires professional advice and supervision throughout the cycle. Discussing each in detail is well beyond this book, but know that they have all been around for decades and there is a lot of information out there if you look hard enough.

A more recent introduction to the bodybuilding scene is injectable Human Growth Hormone (HGH). Literally the hormone that your pituitary gland produces for boys to grow into men. Guys using HGH are easy to spot because they get big swollen bellies where the HGH causes their intestines to grow.

Because of the way they allow your body to add a lot of size, these mass-builder steroids and HGH are suited for Winter Season, when you're trying to add maximum muscle-mass (at the expense of a little fat gain too).

Anavar/Oxandrolone

The other anabolic steroid that comes up a lot in research is Oxandrolone (original brand name of Anavar). This is a steroid that doesn't promote as much muscle growth in the same way as Dianabol, but it does encourage your body to burn body fat quicker and makes you a bit stronger.

This makes it suitable for bodybuilders in Raiding Season, when they're focussing on cutting fat but maintaining muscle mass.

Oxandrolone is mostly in the form of an oral tablet, meaning it comes with all of the risks of liver damage as other oral steroids. However, because it is lower in hepatotoxicity than oral dianabol or winstrol, it's often referred to as "safer". It's popular however (also with female bodybuilders and female bikini competitors) because it has hardly any of the other side-effects associated with "harder" anabolic steroids.

Why Am I Talking About Steroids?

To be honest, the only reason I wanted to include this section in the book is simply thus:

Almost every professional bodybuilder and fitness personality on Instagram are using anabolic steroids.

This is crucially important for you to remember for one simple reason - so you stop comparing your "natty" results to these guys. If you aren't injecting steroids, you are seriously unlikely to ever get as big or ripped as these guys.

It's okay to idolize your favorite fitness personality, as long as you are honest with yourself about it. Even if he claims to be natural, he has to say this so that he doesn't lose his sponsorship from the supplements companies who want you to think that buying their brand of Whey Isolate will mean you can grow as big as him (often they're fully aware of the steroids, it's as if everyone just pretends not to know).

When you accept this, you start to feel a lot better about the gains you're making as a *Natty* Modern Viking.

Health Risks

Up until now I've spoken mostly on the benefits of steroids - thats because there are lots of great benefits of steroids. I'd argue that if Vikings had steroids available, 100% of them would have been using them!

However, as a Modern Viking you really need to consider the wider implications, and particularly the health sacrifices you're making.

According to WebMD, the side effects of abusing anabolic steroids include:

- Reduced sperm count
- Shrink the testicles
- Hair loss & acne
- Enlarging of your breasts

- High blood pressure (which increases the risks of heart attacks and strokes)
- Liver disease and possibly an increase risk of liver cancer
- Effects on your mood (increased aggression, delusions, addiction)

Another risk of using any of these substances is the lab where you sourced the drug. If you're obtaining the drugs illegally, you don't really have any guarantee about what you're actually taking. There are no FDA or equivalent standards body looking after you. Lab conditions could be poor and unsafe or even worse, the lab may knowingly be selling you a cheaper drug (i.e., Dianabol) and selling it to you as a more expensive drug (i.e., Oxandrolone).

As I emphasized at the beginning of this chapter, abusing anabolic steroids is illegal and dangerous and comes with loads of risks.

Viking Style

Beards

While I'm not going to say that every Modern Viking should grow a beard... at the same time I am. And here's why.

Beards make you feel manly as fuck.

In a recent survey of 1,000 men in New York by Braun, 53% said they felt more attractive just because of their beard. 41% said they felt more confident just because of their beard. And 77% of the men in the survey who didn't have a beard said the only reason they didn't have one was because they couldn't grow one yet!

Viking men would famously grow out their beards, and they took great care of them too. Archeologists regularly find beard jewelry for tying braids into beards, and we know Viking men would wash their beards with lye soap to help dye it blonder.

Growing a beard is a commitment that takes time and patience, as with most Modern Viking transformations. It might take years to get the "full beard" you want, depending on your age and genetics. And you should accept that your ancestors have already done most of the work in deciding what your beard is going to look like.

However, a Modern Viking isn't totally powerless.

Firstly, you should invest in a high quality beard oil. This solves the complaint that comes up 95% of the time about growing a beard - itchiness.

With a daily application of beard oil, this itchiness disappears within a day or two. The oil not only makes the beard feel soft and smell nice, it also helps to promote the beard to grow thicker and quicker.

Secondly, you should visit a professional barber who works with beards. This is easy in most inner cities. It sounds a little metrosexual, but the difference between a properly cut beard and a "home job" is huge. Modern Vikings don't want to look like homeless men of the forest, we still have to look great for our women and look neatly groomed for our day jobs.

Spending a few bucks every month or two will mean that as your beard grows out, it's always looking at its best possible also quite importantly, the barber will be able to properly compliment your jawline with your beard.

One word of caution - when asked, most women in Western culture will say that stubble or a very short beard is far more attractive than a full beard. In fact in a recent survey, only 1% of women said they found a full long beard the most attractive grooming choice!

However, becoming a Modern Viking isn't about pleasing women. It's about making you feel great. And you should take courage in the fact that those 1% of women *really* want to jump on a guy with a full beard, because they don't have many guys to choose from! There are far too many accountants and lawyers who will never be able to achieve that full Modern Viking beard look that you can - so go out there and own that niche market!

Wardrobe Essentials

Men are extremely lucky in that we can re-invent our entire wardrobe with only a handful of items.

My recommended Modern Viking 'look' is no different. It's grounded in a few simple principles:

- Keep it practical
- Keep it well fitted
- Keep it high quality

I used to have 2 full wardrobes of clothes. Everything from cheap t-shirts to expensive dress shirts. I had clothes that I only wore every so often, clothes that I wore every day, and clothes that I never wore anymore.

Hanging on to all of this shit was stopping me from having any sense of style.

The first thing I did as a Modern Viking was throw away any impractical clothes - the stuff that looked OK but was just uncomfortable to wear and move in. Life is too short to spend it feeling uncomfortable.

Second was throwing away all of the baggy clothes - the ones that were comfortable as hell, but my female and gay friends told me they made me look like a moody teenager. When a grown man wheres baggy clothes, you project an image of low confidence, low status and low self-esteem.

Clothes should be as close a fit as possible without being uncomfortable. Wearing a tailor-fit blazer jacket and closer fitted dark jeans is one of the best ways to instantly upgrade your outfit.

Invest in a pair of high quality brown leather boots (Modern Vikings never wear black leather). Boots have a strange way of making men feel more masculine, and one pair of brown leather boots is going to go with almost everything else in your wardrobe.

After that it's all about personal choice.

Avoid t-shirts as much as possible - the only time to wear a t-shirt is when you're going to the gym. Try and stay with collared shirts, invest in 2 for casual and 2 for evenings out. Now that you're going to be putting on muscle mass, shirts are going to fit you so much better and really show off the manly "V" taper that you have now.

Stick to dark jeans and pants. Simple and masculine items that are understated, but classy. Always choose to buy 1 pair of $80 jeans over 2 pairs of $40 jeans - not for the brand or anything like that, but because you feel so much better wearing a pair of great fitted jeans every day than owning 2 pairs of jeans that don't make you feel *great*.

Hair Grooming

Growing your hair out long like a Viking is a choice (one I'm making). But you don't need to.

Award winning San Francisco and New York salon hair stylist Jefferson Mosquera (yeah, my hair guy and best friend) says:

"The most important thing is to keep enough length on the top that a woman can run her hands through it. But keep it as short and close on the sides as possible - for most men this emphasizes a masculine face shape and helps to make the face seem slimmer."

When I asked him about grooming products and how a Modern Viking can look neat without risking looking too feminine, his advice was this:

"Stick to high quality pomades and waxes - they seem expensive at first but they last a lot longer. Never buy cheap gels or hair products, they quickly look bad and stop a woman from wanting to get her hands into your hair!"

My advice among anything is to visit the most expensive barber/salon you can afford. Once I stopped getting my $5 haircut and started getting a less regular, but better quality $40+ hair cut, I noticed my hair was easier to style and I could for the most part just forget about it.

This was because the style had already been "cut in" and I knew that I didn't need to worry about trends or fashions, that was my stylists job. He knew I was a straight guy who wanted to look masculine, he knew the shape of my face and the type of hair I had, and he gave me the best style that was right for me and would look 'on-trend'.

Viking Mindset

Confidence

Confidence is the feeling of having absolute faith in your own abilities or values. It means you know that you've got this. You're confident you'll win the battle. You're confident the ship won't sink. You're confident your Damascus Steel sword won't break when it meets the inferior Saxon steel.

As a Modern Viking, confidence is one of the most important goals we're trying to achieve. Almost everything in this book is aimed around improving your own confidence. Sometimes consciously, other times subconsciously.

One of the most common associations with masculinity is confidence - ask any man what makes another man masculine and you'll hear the word confident thrown in there. Ask any woman who says she wants a manly man what that actually means, and pretty quickly you'll hear the word confidence.

When you're confident, life becomes better. Clothes look better. Your sex life becomes better. Your financial health becomes better. The relationships with your family become better.

Confidence is something that is both caused by positive experiences, and also becomes the cause of positive experiences.

This means the achievement of an increased confidence is not absolute - you don't have it or don't have it. In some situations you'll feel more confident than in others. You could feel extremely unconfident in your salsa classes, yet extremely confident in the gym.

You might feel very confident approaching a beautiful woman on the street while she's enjoying a coffee alone on a sunny terrace, yet feel extremely unconfident about approaching the same beautiful women in a lounge bar.

Confidence Makes You Feel Good

You may have set out on your journey to become a Modern Viking for various reasons, but if you are anything like me, it's because you want to increase the amount of happiness in your life.

Happiness comes from many sources and many things, but one of the biggest sources of happiness is an increased confidence.

When you're more confident in yourself, you have few insecurities, fewer self-doubts, and are able to enjoy more situations to their fullest.

Confident people volunteer for opportunities. Confident people get involved in the conversation of the group. Confident people introduce themselves to more people and therefore meet more interesting people.

When you increase your confidence, your happiness increases.

When you imagine Vikings as strong fierce warriors, you miss half of the story. When they weren't on the battlefield or getting on with the mundanity of life (fishing, farming , etc.), Vikings were busy enjoying life.

A Viking would have no problem with standing up in his Lords feasting hall and bursting out into song in front of 40 of his brothers. A Viking has no problem with stripping naked and swimming naked in the river to the laughter of his brothers. A Viking has no problem in throwing his woman over his shoulder and making a game of carrying her to his bed!

The Sagas speak of Vikings as extremely extroverted people, confident in their ability to live life and to make the most of situations.

As a Modern Viking, you can continue to embrace this confident approach to the experiences and opportunities that life presents you with. You may not always have the maximum confidence in the situation (and we'll discuss how to improve that later), but you should know that a bounteous hoard of happiness awaits you if you're willing to embrace your confidence and throw yourself into life!

Confidence Is Feeling Able, Competence Is Being Able

As you increase your confidence, you're going to be projecting to the outside world (and inwards to yourself) that you have faith and conviction in your ability to perform well.

When you act confident at your salsa class, you're telling all the other women in the class that you're a good salsa dancer. When you act confident in a bar, you're telling other women in the bar that you're a good conversationalist. When you act confident in your job interview, you're telling the interviewer that you're good at the job they're hiring for.

Acting confident in situations that require skill is how humans tell other people that they're good at that skill.

However… here's the kicker - there's no real connection between confidence (feeling able) and competence (being able). It's entirely possible to act 100% confident in situations where you have no competence. In fact, it's usually the best way to approach a new situation where you want to start working on your competence.

Embracing this difference, and accepting that the two are not linked as closely as you'd think, is one of the first steps in increasing your confidence. Because when you realize that you don't have to be great at talking to women yet to appear confident at the bar, you remove a huge barrier of self doubt that could be preventing you from genuinely *being* confident. When you realize that not all of the confident people in your salsa class are actually any good at salsa, you're able to start embracing an increased confidence yourself.

And as we know, when we feel more confident, we're able to extract more happiness and enjoyment from a situation.

Once you're able to throw yourself more into the situation through your increased confidence, you'll be exposing yourself to the activity itself more and be able to actually practice it, enjoy it, and become better at it. You'll be able to start working towards mastery.

Confidence Through Mastery

One of the pillars of masculinity is mastery. As I discussed in the introduction, a man's ability to be accepted into the tribe relied hugely on his skills and abilities that he brought into the tribe. This held true for Vikings and it holds true for Modern Vikings today.

If a Viking had excellent combat skills and could always be relied on to hold a strong shoulder, then men would want to stand next to him in the shield wall. He would be respected and people knew he could be relied upon. He had achieved a state of mastery in battle - which gave him a huge amount of confidence when he stood on the battlefield. He had confidence in his own abilities, which means he would be less likely to feel fear, anxiety, worry. Maybe he'd even be able to feel a degree of happiness.

But away from the battlefield, when back in the village, even if the task or scenario he was engaged in wasn't anything to do with combat, that confidence from his mastery will follow him.

Particularly if the same people are around him and involved in the same activity. Because when you achieve confidence from genuine mastery in something valuable, you're able to feel more confident in yourself in other situations.

As a Modern Viking, one of the best ways to give an all around boost to your confidence in all situations is to focus in on one or two of your skills and interests and work towards mastery in that skill area.

This doesn't mean becoming a "little bit good" at tennis, or a "better than average" swimmer. Every man has the potential in him to become truly great at something, and you need to discover this inner skill.

In his revolutionary Bestseller 'Outliers', Malcolm Gladwell proposes that achieving true mastery into a skill requires 10,000 hours of dedication[14]. This means years. Years of working on the same skill, on becoming the top 1% of people in that area.

---

[14] http://gladwell.com/outliers/the-10000-hour-rule/

It may seem like a ridiculous use of your time - perhaps you're thinking I'm talking bullshit. But the theory is sound and my own experiences of working towards mastery for an increased confidence have held true.

I have spent most of my teenage and adult life, on and off, training martial arts. Some of that time has been largely wasted - when I trained Capoeira for example. I didn't take it seriously and unsurprisingly, I didn't become very good and it didn't make me feel the slightest bit better about myself.

But when I switched my attention to Kickboxing, and dedicated 4+ years of my time towards it, I started to become quite good. I started to feel confident, especially when I was around other people who knew me as a good kickboxer. But even when I wasn't, I knew that I wasn't just good at something, I was great. I was better than a lot of people, and I was on my way to being better than most people.

You don't have to go out and become the best boxer, kick boxer or MMA fighter to feel confident from mastery. This is just my example. Mastery over physical skills is an extremely Viking endeavor, but your skills and interests can be about pretty much anything, as long as you become great at it.

If you want to be the best goddam hair stylist on the West Coast, as you work towards it and start becoming better than a lot of other stylists, then better than most stylists, and then after 5-10 years, one of the best stylists, you're guaranteed to have an immense amount of confidence that will sit with you in all situations. It won't mean that you'll instantly become the most confident when in the gym, or the most confident when approaching women, but you'll start with a much higher baseline thanks to your mastery.

Faking Confidence

A common tactic advised by life coaches and well meaning friends is to "fake it until you make it".

It's a great idea to feel confident about something that you don't yet have a great competence in. As I discussed in the previous section, this is one of the best ways to ensure you throw yourself into new situations fully and get happiness from them almost immediately.

However, you can't fake the confidence. You can fake the competence (i.e., through a high confidence) but faking the confidence won't work.

It's a subtle difference, but makes all the difference.

People who fake confidence simply run through the tactics and mannerisms associated with confident people. They force themselves to hold confident posture. They force themselves to demonstrate confident body language. They force themselves to dive into the situation even though they are feeling petrified and massively uncomfortable.

The problem with this is that people are going to eventually see through it. And when we see someone who is faking confidence, we instinctively know this person is massively unconfident. It's much better to express your genuine confidence in a situation, even if it's only middle confident, than to fake a huge amount of confidence that will be shattered once someone calls you out on it.

You may still be wondering what the difference is between genuinely feeling confidence, especially in situations where you don't have competence, and faking the confidence (which you now know is bad).

The key difference is that genuine confidence comes from your Mindset.

If you allow the genuine confidence to come from your subconscious, from the way you think and approach a situation, then your body will follow. You will express yourself as a confident person, you'll stand and talk and act like a confident person.

However, if you try and do those things in the hope that your Mindset will catch up, it just won't happen. Confidence must come from inside, from how you feel. You need to know how to feel confidence from within - and as with all of the Mindset work in Modern Viking, it's simply a skill that can be practiced and learned.

Achieving A Confidence Mindset, When You Aren't Confident

When you're in a situation where you feel low confidence, you need to be able to predict confidence out from your Mindset.

The simplest way I've found to do this is using self-affirmations and mantras, speaking them to myself whenever I feel my confidence starting to dip in a situation. This allows me to boost my positive thoughts.

My goal is to consciously connect to how I'm feeling right now, to become aware of the negativity and become aware of the positivity, and then I'll feed the positivity while allowing the negativity to shrink.

To become aware of the negativity, I'll say to myself (in my head) the causes of the fears or insecurities that I'm feeling which I think are the cause of my lack of confidence.

In a bar for example, these might be:

- *"I think those 2 girls over there are giggling at how tall and cumbersome I look"*
- *"That large group of guys think I'm a loser because I'm alone"*
- *"The bartender is waiting to see me get rejected by those girls"*
- *"I'm over dressed for this bar. I'm wearing a tailored jacket but most of the guys in here are wearing simple t-shirts"*

Once I'm aware of each fear or anxiety bothering me, I'll then run through the best case scenario of each one and start to embrace the fact that I'm being far too harsh on myself:

- *"Those 2 girls are probably talking about how cute I look and are blushing because I looked over"*
- *"The bartender sees guys chat up women 100 times a night. He's not paying the slightest bit of attention to me"*
- *"The large group of guys probably wish they had the confidence to go into a bar alone, and I bet they all wish they were 6'5" like me"*
- *"All of the guys in here wish they shopped in a store for adults like I did, and all the women probably see me as a more sophisticated gentleman compared to the rest of the 'brah!' guys in here"*

We're often too critical of ourselves, but when we become conscious of the negativity within us, we can begin to starve it of our energy and feed the positivity inside us instead.

With this activity, I'm literally talking to myself in my head.

"Liam, those girls probably think you're cute. You are better dressed than most guys in here. You have a better physique than most guys in here. It takes a confident guy to come into a bar alone. That group of guys are probably really fun guys to hang out with"

When you feed the positive thoughts in your mind, the confidence begins to show through. Those mannerisms and side effects of a confident person that we discussed earlier start to naturally and genuinely show through. People in the situation start to see you as a confident person. And then with the confidence, you feel happy, you want to throw yourself into the situation. You want to start talking to women, or you want to make new friends and chat with that group of guys. You have the confidence of a charismatic and interesting guy in the bar and then you become able to get out there and start practicing that skill so that it becomes true.

This technique is basically 'Mindfulness for Beginners'. Become aware of how you're feeling, good and bad, and start to feed the positivity while being aware off the negativity but allowing it to become naturally subdued.

Confidence And Style

While you may think of Vikings as dirty barbarians, smeared in the blood of their enemies and styling themselves in the primal masculinity of dirt and the real world, the reality was quite different.

Vikings, particularly Viking men and warriors, were extremely conscious of their image and their style. Vikings would wash their hair with bleaching soap to maintain bright blonde hair, they would have servants spend hours braiding intricate styles and designs into their hair and beards, and they were extremely fond of jewelry.

In fact, one of the most important symbols of Viking warrior status were Arm Rings, bracelets of precious metal that were worn as a symbol of your manhood, status and wealth. Your first arm ring would be given to you by the lord that you swore an oath to, and then subsequent arm rings would be earned in battle as plunder. The most prominent warriors of the battle would be entitled to take the most arm rings from the enemies they killed.

A Viking lord of war could be seen wearing as many as 5 arm rings on each arm, a statement to his enemies that he had killed many other important men in battle and to face him would be to challenge a great warrior.

As a Modern Viking, you should be aware of your own style as a matter of confidence and as a symbol of your status and mastery.

All women will testify that a confident man with a great sense of fashion is already over 50% of the way to looking attractive, if not even more.

However, what you may not realize is how closely connected confidence and sense of style are.

When famous Hollywood actors are photographed grabbing a Pumpkin Latte on a lazy Sunday afternoon, wearing simple slacks and a plain t-shirt, they still look great. Why is that? It's because of their confidence (and a few hidden tricks about those "simple" clothes).

When a famous actor goes to his local coffee shop, he knows he's richer than most men he will cross paths with. He knows he's a better actor (mastery) than most men he will cross paths with. He knows he has a beautiful wife/girlfriend and he knows that with a small amount of effort, he can make himself look so attractive that photographers will snap him and put him on the cover of their magazine for women to swoon over.

He has such a huge amount of confidence that emanates from his Mindset, that whatever he wears, he will look great.

(He's also helped a little by the fact that his simple t-shirt is probably tailored to cut exactly to his torso, and those simple slacks were tailored to exactly emphasize his silhouette. Don't underestimate how important complimentary fit is in men's fashion!)

When you go out of the house with a huge sense of confidence in yourself, your sense of style just looks better. And when your style looks better, you start to feel more confident. The two feed into each other.

Being Confident Alone

One of the most intimidating situations for guys to face, and one if the most difficult situations to increase your confidence, is being alone in social settings.

Drinking alone in a bar, eating lunch alone in a cafe, turning up to an evening reception alone.

With age, men tend to naturally become more confident in these situations, pretty much because they've naturally acquired a sense of Zero Fucks Given by that point.

But it sucks to spend your 20's and 30's feeling unable to do stuff like this alone.

When I was younger, I would never go to anything without my fiancée or my brothers. If no one was free to meet me for lunch, I would eat at my desk. If no one was free to go for a drink, I would stay home.

This sucked for two reasons:

I missed out on a lot of potentially great experiences and meeting awesome people

Once those people were no longer in my life, I wasn't able to attend any social situations anymore

One of the first things I had to learn when I started traveling as a Digital Nomad was how to feel comfortable and confident alone. After spending over 5 years of always having my fiancé and best friend by my side, I'd literally forgotten how to be alone. And before and after meeting her, every time I'd ever approached a girl in a bar had been as part of a group of friends.

All of my confidence came from being around people. Which is natural - Tribes are a huge part of our lives and going into situations with a strong group of trusted brothers can greatly increase our enjoyment of it.

However, I needed to learn how to feel comfortable alone as well. Mostly because I had no choice if I was going to go out and meet new people!

As with confidence Mindset work, most of the anxiety and apprehension we feel about being alone is irrational - it's the negative wolf in our head trying to see the worst in every situation. Just as before, you need to feed the positive wolf, assume the best, and tell yourself the things you need to hear so that you can enjoy the situation.

With that said, there are a few things worth mentioning for Modern Vikings who want to go adventuring as a lone warrior:

Most men, at some point in their lives, have eaten or drank alone in a bar. You are not a loner and you are not the odd one out. You may feel that other guys sitting in groups are judging you but honestly, they haven't even noticed you! No one cares that you're alone because most people are busy enjoying their own evening. This is something I quickly learned at conferences - everyone comes alone. It's OK. Everyone is there to network and meet new people, so be the confident Viking and say hello to as many people as possible!

Women respond very strongly to social proof (social status is a huge component of attraction), which means having the validation and approval of other people. If you go to a bar alone, you should make a point of talking with the bartender, door security staff and door promoter as soon as possible. Have you ever wondered why club promoters always seem to be sleeping with lots of beautiful women? It isn't (only) because the girls want free access and free bottles... It's because they're genuinely attracted to guys who seem to know lots of people. Get the point where when you walk in, at least a few guys want to say hello to you, shake your hand , etc. This is much easier if you make a point of hitting the same clubs and bars repeatedly.

If you eat at a restaurant alone, make a point of learning the names of the waiting staff, make conversation and be friendly. Honestly, no one will care that you're eating alone unless you're in a really fancy "date" restaurant. (I've had after-shift drinks with lots of people who work in restaurants this way while traveling.)

It's ok to say hello to groups of people and if they seem like cool people, ask to hang out with them. Don't be pushy or needy (particularly if you have zero social proof) but this is how adults get to know new people.

For a recent example, yesterday while I was writing at the beach in Barcelona, a group of guys who were drinking and sunbathing near to me asked me what I was working on. We struck up a conversation and I ended up spending the evening hanging out with them after work. They were cool guys - as most people are.

Have something to do. Honestly, one of the best ways to feel confident with being alone is to have something to do while you're there. This doesn't mean simply sitting and playing with your phone (a habit that's associated with low confidence and nervousness). Have a genuine interest in what you're doing. For example, I often pitch up with my laptop and start writing, and usually people will say hello and ask me what I'm working on. Another favorite is a newspaper or book. The point isn't to engross yourself purely in the activity - you want to be available to say hello to people who might be interesting, but you just want some kind of 'anchor' to make you feel a bit more comfortable.

Confidence Around Women

The most popular area of confidence that men are looking for when they contact me about Modern Viking is to gain more confidence around women. This was me when I was 18 or 19, and it's still a huge part of my desire at the age of 28. And I hope that well into my 50's, I'm still keen to be "the man" around women.

But I've definitely gained perspective, probably at an accelerated pace than most guys, about the importance of "confidence with women". Or more specifically, I used to *chase* women - now I aim to *attract* them. I studied PUA (pick up artists) like Mystery, Styles and Gambler (3 very famous pick up artists) and I believed that if I learned the tricks and tips, I would sleep with more women and then this would give me more confidence around women.

I was chasing the end reward, cutting corners and skipping out the hard work to build any long-term foundations.

Here's the paradox... PUA works. I studied the "Mystery Method" while I was at University. MM is a system of manipulating the psychology of beautiful, but insecure, women by demonstrating high social value within that exact moment. It worked. I had sex with an uncountable number of women because I "tricked" them into my bed. I was a master of "the game" and it was at the height of my "game" that I met and seduced my fiancée (later to become ex-fiancée) - at the time she was one of the most popular and hottest cheerleaders at my University and I have no doubt that without MM, she would never have spoken to me.

Here's the problem with MM though - not once did it increase my confidence around women.

I was having sex with so many beautiful women, women who I approached in bars and clubs "cold" (i.e., with no previous connection or advantage) and persuaded them to have sex with me within hours of meeting me, but I never felt more confident.

Every night when I went to the clubs or bars with my "wingman," I started from zero again each time. Every night I had to build myself back up, I had to rehearse the "routines," scripts of rehearsed conversations and stories that were proven to hook the majority of women into being intrigued and then attracted to me.

PUA worked to get me more sex, but it didn't work to make me more confident.

Fast forward a few years later and I'd been dumped by my fiancée, I was a single guy, not naturally very attractive, basically broke, and in cities where no one knew me. I had no friends and therefore no social proof. My 'game' was zero all over again.

Apart from I did have something. I had Modern Viking. I had a Zero Fucks Given attitude. I was comfortable sitting in bars alone. I had started to practice a hybrid bodybuilding-strongman weightlifting routine and was eating like a beast. I had grown a beard to help me feel manly as fuck and I was growing my hair long, despite the fact that less than 3% of women find long hair attractive.

And I walked into cafes, terraces, bars, beaches, practiced zero game, and yet had more confidence around women than I'd ever had in my life. I even attracted women who came and approached me!

Sure, this confidence didn't bring me the onslaught of Hollywood-actor-level sex that practicing PUA had. But I felt happy. I felt confident. I enjoyed being around women, in talking with them, in finding out who they were and what their dreams and ambitions were and in building real connections. And I felt extremely confident in telling a woman I did not want to have sex with her! Imagine, feeling so sure in yourself that you don't want to have sex with a woman who is offering it!

For the first time in my life (seriously) I had female friends. More specifically, I'm friends with beautiful women, the type of women who get paid to drink in VIP areas of clubs, but behind the scenes are studying a Masters in Civil Engineering or writing a 100,000 word sci-fi novel. PUA will never give you that, and I can promise you, it's much more fulfilling.

Giving Zero Fucks

Things used to be simple. Catch food. Kill enemies. Fuck women. Try not to die.

But things got more complicated. You have a cell phone. You have cholesterol. You have laws. You have a job.

The luxuries of modern life present you with a plethora of opportunities and rewards, but also with problems, expenses and things demanding your attention.

When we have so much to gain and so much to lose, we start worrying. We start to care. We start *giving fucks*.

Blissfully Ignorant Childhoods

Giving fucks is something you've been doing since you were a child. When you cried because your socks didn't match, when you screamed because your brother got more chicken on his plate than you, when you punched Drew Harrison in his fat stupid face because Lisa Smith kissed him behind the bushes on the school field and not you (true story. Fuck you Drew and fuck you Lisa).

As children, you gave a fleeting fuck about many things. You handed out a piece of your soul to every possible new experience in your day and in return, you were occasionally rewarded with disappointment, heartbreak, envy and sadness.

A broken toy or a bruised knee could seriously fucking ruin your day!

However, you gave zero fucks about the way you looked when you played with worms and beetles. You gave zero fucks if you smelled like garbage because you'd discovered a dead mouse by the trash. You gave zero fucks about dressing up like Spiderman and walking around your local shopping mall. You lived in the moment and life was just one big adventure!

Then you grew up and started to give some semi-serious fucks. You started to comb your hair. You started to shower. You started to care about what you looked like in the mall and you started to care about girls. You started giving even more fucks and as a result, you probably got your heart broken a few times and had some pretty shitty days.

But at that time, you still gave zero fucks about paying the rent. You gave zero fucks about curing cancer. You gave zero fucks about a career. You gave zero fucks about your credit score. You gave zero fucks about your business email.

And then suddenly, you became an adult and started giving fucks bout *everything*.

Everything became a source of worry or disappointment. You cared about your image in public. You worried over finances and your mounting credit card debts. You fretted over where you would find your next sexual encounter. You worried about how many of your colleagues liked you. You started to feel disappointed that your career hadn't gone the way you expected. You worried about whether you looked stupid singing karaoke.

If you think back to those times as a young child, or those times as a teenager, when you gave zero fucks about many things, you might be able to remember the sheer bliss of Zero Fucks Given.

Of simply not caring what the outside world thought when they looked at you.

Giving zero fucks wasn't about being apathetic or indifferent. It wasn't about living life mildly or 'vanilla'. It wasn't about avoiding scrutiny or opinion.

It was about being totally different and maybe weird, and being totally happy with that.

Giving Zero Fucks As A Berserker

Viking berserkers dove into battle shirtless, swinging a battle axe twice the size of an average weapon and screaming furiously for Odin to greet them in Valhalla. They wanted to land in the afterlife on a mountain of slain enemies. They didn't care about their personal safety - after all, the Gods had already decided if they would live or die.

Berserkers embraced their animalistic spirit and they screamed in the faces of their enemies as they cleaved their axe through flesh and bone.

Berserkers dove in and went for the big wins. Go big or go home, and zero fucks given about which way it goes.

Giving Zero Fucks As A Pagan

Zero fucks given permeated throughout Norse religion, and their opinion of other religions too. When Vikings conquered parts of England, they made no attempt to convert Christians to Paganism. They were content with their own spirituality and religion, but they gave zero fucks about which God their Christian neighbors prayed to.

Jesus was just another God after all.

Vikings were not concerned with worrying about the God that their neighbors or enemies bowed to, and were far more interested in enjoying life and stealing the gold of their enemy. The Viking habit of killing Christian priests in cruel and brutal executions was caused not by a hatred of Christianity, but by a hatred of the constant preaching and attempts of Christian missionaries.

Viking pagans never preached to Christians that they would not feast in Valhalla unless they converted. But, Christian priests were constantly preaching to Pagans that they would go to Hell if they did not convert to Christianity.

Christian priests, for giving too many fucks, were rewarded with executions mimicking those of famous Christian martyr deaths.

When you give zero fucks about what path someone else has chosen, and you choose not to preach to them about their choices, you both get to live a happier life and have less negativity (and bloody executions!) in your life.

Having Something To Give A Fuck About

Thats the thing - when you have something genuinely good, exciting and important in life (aka feasting and fucking) you find yourself giving far less fucks about the small details. Christian's spent so much time condemning "heathens" and living miserable lives because their religion denied them of all of the good stuff in life.

"Don't fuck your neighbor's wife. Don't get drunk. Don't have fun. Don't dance naked around a fire..."

(I'm paraphrasing the Bible but that's the general theme)

When there is no excitement in your life, you start spending way too much time worrying about the small and mundane details.

But when you have genuinely fun and interesting things going on, when you have amazing women and amazing brothers in your life, when you have a genuinely exciting and interesting cause to pursue and campaign for, you start giving far less fucks about the God that your neighbor prays to or the Facebook profile picture of your ex-girlfriend.

Dancing To Your Own Beat

If you're going to embrace a Modern Viking life, you're going to start being a bit different from the people around you. Friends and family might start to think your 'obsession' with working out is unhealthy. They may start telling you how dangerous it is to eat a lot of protein. They might tell you about the article they read in Cosmo Magazine how working out any more than 7 Minutes a day is a waste of time.

You'll start to get a lot of friction and pushback from people who care about you, but don't immediately understand what Modern Viking is about. They might have no scientific education on health, fitness and nutrition, they probably have no real historical education on Vikings beyond Hollywood, and even worse, they're probably unaware of their poor education!

But they'll still feel the need to get involved in your business and start telling you their advice.

One of the things you need to get used to when embracing a Viking Mindset is telling this people one simple line:

"Thank you, but shut the fuck up."

You don't need to convince those around you that your new workout or meal plan is a good idea. It's not your job to educate them. You don't need them to understand the scientific studies backing the effectiveness of daily self-affirmations, for those affirmations to be effective for *you*.

Dancing to your own beat and doing your own thing is going to be an everyday component of being a Modern Viking.

It's good practice - because you're also going to get a much more valuable life and healthier Mindset when you start applying this attitude to other aspects of your life.

When you remove yourself from the judgement of other people, you start being able to enjoy more freedom to do the things you want to do. You gain the freedom to express yourself in whatever way that you want to.

Do you feel like growing a full beard? Fuck what your colleagues think!

Who cares if your friends think cheerleading is for only for gays. Go and join a team and get your back handspring game on!

So your parents think that being a poet is a dumb career choice. Well, maybe they're right, but being an accountant is a suicide-inducing career choice too, so fuck that, go out and start trying to sell your rhymes!

Being weird, if weird is genuinely you (and most of us are a bit weird) is so much fun. Don't deny yourself of the liberating freedom of just being you.

Give Less Fucks About Other People

While maintaining a healthy tribe of brothers and close family is extremely important to a life as a Modern Viking, there's also a lot of people in your life right now who really don't deserve to be there. And one of the worst problems with having so many shit people in your life, is how many fucks they expect you to give (and waste).

Those 'friends' who make you feel uncomfortable about your table-top gaming hobby. Those 'friends' who say that eating bacon is evil. Those 'friends' who tell you that ballet is for snobs and gays.

Fuck those people, and definitely stop giving fucks about their opinions and judgements.

Because when you really think about it, what are the consequences of their opinion? How do their judgements and snide remarks really effect your life?

So they think that your hobby spent painting small plastic miniature models and playing table-top war games makes you a loser. So what? Does that mean your dick suddenly falls off? Does that mean your bank account suddenly resets to $0? Does that mean you no longer get to fuck Sarah on Wednesdays and Claire on Saturdays?

When you realize how little someone's opinion really affects you, you can start giving zero fucks about it.

Giving fucks about people's opinions was a skill we had to learn as children: Learning to dress the same way the popular boys dressed, learning to talk how the popular boys dressed, learning to be good at the same sports the popular boys were good at. These skills have a purpose and are valuable when we're trying to build bonds with brothers, when we want them to feel familiar with us, and we want to be accepted into the group.

But as an adult, your life is totally unaffected by what your friend's girlfriend thinks about your new interest in fitness. Your career will still keep progressing at the same pace despite the fact that the receptionist in your office doesn't like your beard. Your dick will still get sucked this weekend even though your old high school friend on Facebook insisted that supplementing Creatine is bad for your kidneys.

Fuck the insignificant people in your life and the fucks they try to get from you.

Giving Less Fucks About Your Friends' Drama

One huge source of distractions trying to take your fucks is the drama in your friends lives. I'm all for being there for a brother: I'll help you get a new job, I'll help you move house, I'll even help you move a body!

But as a Modern Viking, one area I won't give you any of my fucks, is your exaggerated emotional drama.

If your brother wants to share a sex story from the weekend, great. Have that chat. If your brother wants to tell you about the free food and beer available in his new job, great. Have that chat.

But if your brother wants to moan about how his girlfriend doesn't blow him as often anymore, and how she's struggling with her diet and it's causing them to fight, and she earns a bit less money than him and they're fighting over splitting bills... and drama... and drama... and more drama.

You just need to give zero fucks about that drama.

Your own life has enough drama with people close to you, all demanding you give them some of your fucks. Your mum and dad are having issues and you're trying to help your baby sister stay out of the mess, so you take her to ice cream on the weekends and you take her to and from gymnastics practice. That's the sort of drama worth giving fucks about.

When you have the power to directly influence the drama, and it benefits people really close to you, then you should probably give a fuck.

But when the person is simply venting their drama at you, and eventually they're the only person who will be able to go and fix that drama, then what the fuck are they telling you for?

Because they simply want to vent.

Well, I'm sorry but if your brother just wants to vent his crap, he should get a dog. Taking a dog for a walk in the woods and venting your drama to the wind for only your dog to hear, without bothering anyone else, is what a real man does.

Don't burden your brothers with your shit. Don't ask them to give their valuable fucks about your petty shit, and they won't ask the same from you.

Be The Guy Who Gives Zero Fucks

Once you get into the habit of giving zero fucks, your brothers will know this about you. One simple glaring stare will tell them that what they're saying right now has zero chance of extracting any fucks from you, and they'll drop the subject.

Don't be a total dick, but make it clear so that they know your fucks are valuable and what they're complaining about is not worth one of them. Become known as the Modern Viking who is there when people need him, who is ready to jump into battle with axe swinging, who is ready to raid and pillage and plunder when you want him… but only when you *really* need him to give a fuck.

As people get used to your zero fucks given attitude, they'll stop judging your outfit, your hobbies, your choices, and they'll start to admire and respect you for it.

"Oh my god, did you hear Dave told his boss to shove the new dress code up his ass? Dave is the man, he gives zero fucks!"

"Oh there goes Dave again, what is that suit he's wearing? He looks like he's about to go on stage as a standup comedian! Wow Dave gives zero fucks!"

"Did you hear Dave sang 'Let It Snow' last night at the company karaoke? He was such a performer, everyone was laughing and it was awesome! He gives zero fucks!"

People will admire you and respect you and they'll also start to think you're the guy who knows how to have fun, the guy who's comfortable and confident in himself, the guy who's a leader worth following.

Insecurities

Modern Vikings Don't Have Time For Insecurities

Insecurities are the enemy of a confident and happy Modern Viking. When you allow yourself to have deep-rooted insecurities, you open your mind to jealousy, low self-esteem and unhappiness, and you're almost guaranteed to push anything amazing in your life away.

This means leaving your insecurities unchecked can put your job, your woman or your friendships at risk. Insecurities may be rooted in truth, i.e., your nose really is that big. Or they may be entirely irrational, i.e., you think blonde hair makes you look like a young boy, but you want to look like a big man! (FYI Most Swedish Vikings were blonde, and the ones who weren't would dye their hair blonde!)

While male insecurities are usually based on physical attributes, there are emotional insecurities as well that may be eroding your confidence from within. These types of insecurities include your performance in bed, your ability to emotionally satisfy your woman, your ability to perform at work or your insecurities about socializing in groups.

Insecurities tend to be long term - they've usually developed over a long period of time and compounded to the point of feeling like it's a constant part of who you are.

But a Modern Viking knows this is bullshit; Everything about you can be improved (well, almost everything. Unfortunately if you're 5'8" then you're pretty much always going to be that height!)

Insecurities From Childhood

So many of the insecurities we have as adults actually started in childhood. The little bastards on the playground were kind enough to point out why you were different. Those little fuckwits were creative enough to think of nicknames for your hairy birthmark, your pointy nose, your weird limp.

But here's the thing - children are mean little shits. You were probably also a mean little shit. Before bullying becomes bullying, it's just name calling. It's highlighting your friends' differences. It's being curious about the differences of the world.

We were all mean little shits… it's just that some little boys and girls got spanked back at home a bit too much, their parents got divorced, their older brothers beat the crap out of them and stole all of their toys, their uncle Jimmy showed them too much attention. So these children evolved from curious name calling into bullying - they were forced to find weaknesses in the other children because they needed control over something in their lives. These poor little kids became the bullies of your older childhood years, when most children had grown out of being a mean little shit.

As an adult, you need to realize that these poor kids and teenagers probably have extremely fucked up lives right now. They probably sit on welfare and have 2,000 Facebook friends in the hope of feeling any genuine connection with people anymore.

The insecurities from childhood that probably still have an annoying place deep in your subconscious were probably planted there by children or teenagers who don't deserve you hate, but instead your sympathy.

Big ass nose? Don't worry, some of the most attractive male celebrities have large noses. It's a proven sign of high testosterone levels.

Bullied for being a lanky freak? Well I was… believe it or not, children used to (try to) bully me for being tall. Then puberty hit, and I grew to be a 6 foot tall 12 year old. And those poor little boys stayed around 5 foot and never grew much taller, and now they're 28 years old, injecting a ton of Anabolic Steroids and paying for a sports car on a Credit Card to try and cover up their insecurities about their height.

I experienced a mild amount of bullying at school, though only partly for my physical appearance. I didn't have any particularly grotesque features and apart from my obscene height and wonky buck teeth (less of an issue in UK as I think it would have been in USA), I don't think I really experienced any bullying of note. But I was socially awkward and weird as fuck, and a bit of an arrogant shit about being smarter than 95% of the children in my class.

So any bullying I got was probably well earned, but I've let go of it years ago using the following techniques.

As with all of your Viking Mindset work, you need to become aware of each insecurity that you have, or had, because of your childhood. Think back to the things that made you unhappy as a small child and as a teenager.

How many of them are you still holding onto?

As I did with my height and my teeth, you need to think rationally about the physical differences that fellow classmates highlighted about you. And then let go of them. Rationalize them as an adult in an adult society. Why are you still refusing to wear shorts on the beach, just because 15 years ago some kids said your birthmark on your calf looked like a shit stain?!

See it from their point of view. Why were they saying that? What did their lives look like at the time? What didn't you know about David's home life? Do you have any idea the shit that Sarah was going through with her parents divorce? Do you honestly think that Suhail and Ishmael weren't getting enough of their own racist shit when they rode 2 buses home, that the only time they could feel a little bit of power was in trying to get a group of children to laugh at your fat lard ass during sports?

Kids are mean little shits. They're mean little shits because they're in constant emotional turmoil, trying to make sense of the world, their bodies, their family, society... Let go of the negative baggage that you're still carrying from your childhood, no matter how minor you may think it is.

Physical Insecurities You Can't Do Anything About

As a Modern Viking, you already know the importance of building a strong and muscular body. You're already correcting your fashion and your style. You're already working towards being more socially confident and charismatic.

But there are going to be things about your body that you can't change. It's simply who you are.

You're not going to grow any taller. Your skin is always going to be that color. Your nose isn't going to change shape. Your dick isn't going to get any bigger.

(Actually, your dick is going get a tiny bit bigger. Your erections get slightly thicker and harder once you lower your body fat and increase your cardiovascular health thanks to increased blood flow. This mainly applies to guys who were obese before, however I personally noticed the difference too after coming from around 25% body fat, and girls who had known me before and after Modern Viking commented the same too.)

Unless you're a millionaire and become obsessed with plastic surgery, there are plenty of things about your physical appearance that you just aren't going to change. And the sooner you become aware of, and accept these differences, the sooner you can own them. Once you own them, you can let go of them as weaknesses and insecurities, and embrace them as who you are.

I am very tall. You might be very short. But you might have a beautiful Hollywood smile, whereas mine looks like a rabbit got raped by Prince William. You might not have a huge 'locker room dick' but a distinctively average 'party time dick'. You might be muscular but have tiny calves.

When you own your physical insecurities, they quickly lose the power to hurt you or lower your self esteem. When you embrace that they aren't going to change no matter how much attention you pay them, you quickly realize it's wasted attention and you can focus on other things.

Insecurities In A Relationship

Once you've embraced your physical insecurities - the ones you can change and get rid of, and the ones that are just part of who you are - then you can move onto dealing with your emotional insecurities and the ones that are affecting your mindset from within.

One of the main areas that most Modern Vikings want to work on is the insecurities in their relationship.

When a man allows insecurities to take hold of him in a relationship, it inevitably results in the woman leaving him or even worse, cheating on him. Insecurities in relationships tend to be self-fulfilling prophecies.

A constant insecure fear of your girlfriend cheating on you has a shitty way of causing her to cheat on you.

When you have a high value woman (as most Modern Vikings want to achieve), a natural instinct is to want to protect that. She took a lot of game, charming and romance to get to the stage where she lets you bury your axe in her regularly. As a biological animal, it's very easy to become worried about losing her and having to repeat that investment all over again.

However, this is all part of a Fear Of Loss Mindset and your insecurities.

A confident man, certain of his physical, social and emotional value, will feel far less insecure in a relationship with a beautiful woman than an insecure and low esteem guy.

This is easy to identify in yourself - have your last few relationships with women felt like you were "punching above your weight"? Did you friends or her friends make you feel like she was better than you? Did you constantly accuse her of cheating on you, of flirting with colleagues, of texting her male friends too much?

Insecurity in a relationship is a poison and manifests itself as jealousy. Even as the jealousy ebbs and flows, the insecurity within you is constant and will carry with you from relationship to relationship - every time you get an amazing woman, eventually your insecurities will come out and sabotage it. Either very quickly, or as a slow burning poison, depending on the experience of the woman (women who have had insecure boyfriends in the past tend to be experts at spotting it in future guys).

Here's your problem - beautiful and high value women have a lot of options. Even though it isn't in the biological programming for women to be unfaithful (nearly all women are programmed to be monogamous) eventually if you repeatedly demonstrate low value with your insecurity, she will start to look elsewhere. All those secure and confident men who approach her every day swill start to become more appealing!

Getting a Viking Body, becoming charismatic and confident in social situations, getting a great Viking Tribe around you and generally becoming an awesome guy, is all going to count for shit if you allow your insecurities to creep up on you once you're in a relationship.

If you want to keep your amazing woman, you need to conquer those insecurities before it's too late!

Monogamy And Insecurity

To understand insecurity in a relationship, you first need to become aware of and embrace where it comes from.

One of the main sources of insecurity that men feel is the monogamy that's forced upon us by modern society.

Men are told that having sex with more than one partner is bad. You should work hard to seduce one woman, and then once she allows you to fuck her, she's the only woman you should fuck. All ties to other women you had in the pipeline should be broken off and you should focus all sexual energy and attention on this one woman.

I'm not here to call judgement on monogamy or honest polygamy (dishonest polygamy though is fucked up - don't be that guy).

Regardless of your choices, you need to be aware of the effect that monogamy has on you as your evolutionary biology fights against your Mindset.

When you're monogamous, you become fearful of losing that woman. After all, you spent a lot of time seducing her and demonstrating your value to her. If she was to suddenly wake up one morning and leave you, you would have to put in all of that effort again to eventually find another woman of equal or higher value.

Or even worse, you might not find another woman of the same value and have to settle for a woman of lower value!

This mindset is something you need to conquer.

Sure, it's founded partly in truth - going out and getting another woman isn't a walk in the park.

But if you've continued to invest in yourself and never became complacent during the relationship, then you'll actually be higher value than when you met her. Because improving yourself is a continual process, and as long as you keep moving forwards, you're continually improving.

So embrace this reality - if she leaves you, you will be able to go out and find another high value woman. Your value as a man is only partly based on your looks. Women are far more interested in your confidence, your style, your social status, your financial stability... all attributes that a Modern Viking is continually improving about himself.

It's A Lot Easier For A Woman To Get Laid

A common cause of insecurity for many men in relationships is the simple fact of how much easier it is for a woman to go out and get laid.

A man needs to dress well, workout, have social status and internalize a good confident game to appear charismatic to a woman. Then he needs to put himself out there at bars, meetups, libraries, clubs, parties... he needs to meet many woman and eventually, one of them will be interested in having sex with him.

A woman needs to put on a small black dress, maybe some make up, and go out to the nearest bar. Literally, that's all.

This simple fact of society causes many insecure men to panic and constantly have anxiety.

"If she wants to, she could go and fuck another man tonight!"

Here's the tough love brother: that's totally true. She could. But that doesn't mean she will.

(But sometimes, they do.)

I've had fights with girls who have stormed out, and literally within a few hours, have sent me photos of themselves in bed with a hot guy (Yes, I've dated some crazy bitches).

That's just the risk when you aim high and you get a high value woman - you set yourself up for this possibility. But let's play out that scenario - who actually wins/loses?

She goes out and walks to the front of a VIP queue at a trendy bar. Within 15 minutes she's drinking $500 bottles and laughing and joking with a bunch of finance guys. 2 hours later, his cum is dripping out of her and onto his $750 silk bedsheets. He's fast asleep because he needs to be at his desk for 7.30am and she's Snapchatting photos of herself in bed with him to send to you.

Do you think she honestly feels like she 'won' tonight? Does she feel loved by the new guy? Does she feel a genuine connection? Does she still feel high value?

A man's insecurities about a woman going out and getting 'instant sex' comes from how you project your own opinion of sex on to hers.

Women (rarely) desire physical attraction and sexual gratification in the same way men do. For a woman to enjoy a sexual connection, she needs to be intrigued by the man, she needs to be seduced, she needs to be made to feel safe and secure, she wants to feel an emotional connection etc. (There's another 947 other variables that I'm still figuring out).

Whereas a man is simply happy if the woman has a nice pair of tits, a small waist and a round ass!

Women and men are satisfied by a sexual connection in different ways. If a man goes out and gets a quick one night stand, it's high fives all round. If a woman does it, she probably won't feel fully satisfied.

And I'm not in any way talking about social "slut shaming" or satisfied in terms of being able to orgasm. It's simply about how men and women rate sexual encounters and what we desire from them.

So back to my scenario (which has unfortunately happened more than once). The girl storms out, and tries to hurt me, or show her dominance, whatever… by hooking up with a guy within a few hours. But I know she feels no connection, I know her satisfaction lasted only a few minutes, and I know she feels cheap.

Meanwhile, I spent the last few hours playing some Xbox, reading a new research study on Glutamine, and talking to some friends about the upcoming weekend's plans.

Does my apathy mean I'm cold and don't care? In a way - yes. I don't care that she went out and got instant sex because I know most women can go out and get easy sex. And with a good guy too - there are many wealthy and good looking guys in clubs who are experts at taking home women who are on the rebound from their boyfriends.

I've rationalized the situation and considered what's really happening. I've become aware and mindful of how her actions make me feel. I'm also not insecure about my own ability to attract a new high value woman, and enjoy a meaningful sexual connection with her.

As with many negative influences on your Viking Mindset, the first step is to become aware of it. Accept that this possibility is bothering you (if it is).

Become conscious of your subconscious insecurities that your woman could go out and have sex with another man very easily. Become aware of the possibility that the 5 or 6 times a day when men flirt with her (and they do, whether she tells you or not), she could easily say yes and hand over her phone number.

And then rationalize it to yourself. Play out the worst case scenario. What are the consequences, what are the costs, how will your life and happiness really be affected?

Once you've analyzed the worst case scenario - so you know the risks at stake, then run through the chances that this would actually happen.

Have you been acting like a Modern Viking in the relationship? Are you taking care of yourself, building a strong Viking Body? Do you make her feel safe and secure? Does your positive Viking Mindset allow you to also connect to her emotions in a positive way?

Do you regularly pick her up, carry her to the bedroom, and fuck her senseless as if <u>Ragnarök</u> was just around the corner?

If you're doing these things, you're probably giving your high value woman everything she needs in the relationship and there's little to no reason why she'd need to go out and sexually explore another man.

Once you've realized that this is not going to happen, you can let the feelings shrink within you. They won't disappear, and thats ok, but you can spend the energy saved from worrying about it and invest it into enjoying the time with your woman.

Insecurity From Sexual Performance

One of the most common insecurities that many men have is their sexual performance. This could be from an insecurity about the size of your equipment, your ability to last long enough, your ability to make the woman orgasm, or the amount of semen you produce.

Firstly, when it comes to the size of your hammer, you should refer to the section about physical features that you can't do anything about. The cock you have now is what you've got to work with. No reinforcements, no upgrades.

Another insecurity affecting men, particularly emerging in the last few years, is insecurities about the amount of semen you produce during sex. Thanks to the copious amounts of porn we all watch, we've been led to believe that showering a woman in a boatload of your warrior juice is normal.

Here's the reality guys - most of the time, you're watching Methyl-cellulose F50 squirted on her face (interestingly, also the same product used in the Ghostbuster movies for green slime)[15].

The average amount of Viking Venom produced per raid is between a teaspoon and a tablespoon.

So the next time you've got her on her knees and she's begging you to fulfill her porn star fantasy, accept the fact that while she might want a showering, she's more likely to just feel a few drops.

---

[15] https://en.wikipedia.org/wiki/Methyl_cellulose#Special_effects

Another common sexual insecurity, probably as common as penis size, is endurance during sex. Worrying about how quickly you like to win the battle is something that all men have felt at one point, and it's something that tends to stay with you from partner to partner and is often compounded by the mental anxiety of it.

I remember the first time I ever felt like I didn't last long enough - up until that point I'd been fine and usually lasted long enough for the woman to orgasm. However, this was my first real drunk one-night stand. And unsurprisingly, despite the fact that I was feeling a small amount of whisky-dick, I still came long before the girl had even come close to peaking.

And the first thing the evil bitch did was complain about it.

Thus firmly planting an insecurity that lasted for the next 6 months, ruining almost every sexual encounter I had during that time.

Eventually I met a girl and was open enough to explain that I was always anxious about lasting long enough. I explained what had happened on that drunken night, and every one night stand since, and that I was just destined to always cum before the woman.

But she was awesome. She helped me to become aware of the situation fully. To explore it from all angles.

The girl had been very drunk, and probably not very turned on. The encounter was rushed, lacking in foreplay and any emotional connection - all ingredients which innocent 18 year old me learned were essential to get a woman to orgasm.

Too many guys allow their insecurity about lasting long enough to try weird numbing creams, thick condoms, or weird dick-strangling tactics to stop them blowing their load. But once you've slept with enough experienced woman who are willing to be honest with you, you discover that most women don't want a typical sexual encounter to last longer than 30 minutes.

Chaffing and soreness starts to set in!

So the secret to "lasting long enough" isn't in holding in your raiders for an hour - it's in getting the woman to orgasm faster. Making sure you feast first, making sure she's comfortable, making sure there's a genuine connection and attraction between you.

There's another, totally separate side to overcoming this insecurity - some women just won't orgasm from intercourse. While it takes an open and honest girl to tell you this, it's something you can be aware of. Don't allow your negative Mindset to take over and assume the worst in the situation - it might not be because you came after 30 minutes. It might just be that she isn't ever going to orgasm from intercourse, and now you've had your pillaging fun, it's time to be a man and feast on your Goddess' fruit.

Insecurity From Repressed Sexuality

A rarely discussed insecurity that many men have is a fear of expressing their repressed sexuality as a man. Not all guys, but most guys will at some point in their lives be horny beasts who can think about nothing other than having sex with as many women as possible.

For some guys this is a phase for a year or two. For other guys it's their teens, 20's, 30's and most of their 40's!

The problem is that society has told us that men who are overly sexual are perverts. Mainstream media tells women to avoid these men as creeps, players and 'dogs'.

Men become fearful of the boundary, of getting it wrong and becoming labelled as a pervert. A label that carries extreme social shame in nearly all societies.

The problem is, when you get some women behind closed doors, they will tell you that they would love nothing other than to be picked up and fucked all over the house by her Viking! (Actually, I'm directly quoting many women from recent personal experience!)

But even behind closed doors, so many guys can become paralyzed by the fear of expressing their sexuality. Frozen and cut off from being honest with themselves.

And as with all other negative mindsets, this can cost you from experiencing amazing opportunities.

Overcoming this mindset is a delicate matter - you need to become mindful and embrace your nature while at the same time using common sense to gauge the situation. Obviously, you can't just drop a crude bomb on a girl you only met 5 minutes ago, but honestly if the vibe is going well and you're feeling the primal tension, it can sometimes be fun to whisper into a girls ear that you want to fuck her so hard that the neighbors are going to need to smoke a cigarette afterwards!

As with many things, women want genuine confidence and genuine raw passion. Don't try and express yourself as a sexual Viking if that's not you. But if it is, embrace it. Obviously use common sense and a measure of decorum, but if the moment is right and the energy is correct, stick a finger up to conservative conversation and allow the woman to meet the primal warrior within you.

Insecurity Vs. Vulnerability

Something so many guys get wrong in relationships is showing vulnerability versus showing insecurity. Vulnerability can be incredibly attractive to a woman once you're in the relationship - showing a private and hidden part of yourself, just for her.

It allows her to feel a deeper and more personal connection with you, something which women love.

Vulnerability is also an extremely charming quality in peer groups. When someone exposes themselves to us with honesty and homily, we naturally warm to that person. We feel like we know them as a closer friend, like they brought us one level closer to them. They trusted us with a small part of their soul and that trust instinctively encourages us to trust the person back in return.

When a Viking admits that his rear is vulnerable in the shield wall, his brothers appreciate his honesty and humility. They cover his back, and they stand strong on his flanks.

But when you express an insecurity in a relationship, or an insecurity to your friends, it's not cute. It doesn't allow people to warm to you.

It annoys them.

People tend to overcompensate for their insecurities, whereas they are simply aware of (and aware of improving) their vulnerabilities. But our insecurities make us act irrationally.

As a Modern Viking, don't be afraid to show your vulnerabilities and weaknesses. Share them with your partner, your friends and colleagues so that they can feel closer to you.

But don't take that as an excuse for layering your insecurities onto those same people. Handle your insecurities using the techniques in this chapter and invest into yourself to conquer them.

Insecurity At Work

A huge area of insecurity affecting many Modern Vikings is the workplace. The feeling of inadequacy and being out of your depth can cause a constant anxiety and stress. And considering that we spend most of our waking lives at work, this can really start to build up and affect who you are.

Sometimes this can be caused by irrational negative thinking - the demons that you've had to conquer so many times already in achieving a strong Viking Mindset.

- Assuming you perform badly despite the fact that there is no evidence to support this
- Assuming that colleagues don't like you, despite the fact that no one has said anything to suggest this
- Assuming that your colleagues are better than you, despite the fact you all keep hitting the same goals and targets

The key is to become aware of how you really feel about your performance and how you really feel about your colleagues. Examine the evidence available to you right now, and become aware of it without extrapolating or filling in any gaps in knowledge.

Sometimes however, your insecurities may have rational causes. You may actually be out of your depth or you may actually have shitty colleagues.

Repeatedly underperforming and missing targets will quickly deteriorate your confidence and cause insecurities to set in. After a while, these insecurities will become self-fulfilling: believing you will miss your quarterly target has a strong chance of actually causing you to miss your quarterly target.

You need to move into a position (in the same company or a new company) that is still a challenge, but is achievable. A Modern Viking needs to be constantly improving to feel fulfilled, but there are only so many utter defeats in a row that you can take.

If you're in a hostile environment with a team who aren't supporting you, and you've already tried to talk with them and genuinely see if the issues are in your negative thinking or in theirs, then it's time to strap on a pair. No matter how great the pay, the company or the opportunity, you need to get out of that team as fast as possible.

The people around us have a huge impact on our Mindset and overall happiness, and considering the volume of time you spend at work, your colleagues will have one of the biggest influences on you.

It's time to pick up you axe and go look for a new tribe. Trying to fix the situation by chatting to your manager is rarely going to work - a poisonous team already has the sort of culture you don't want to be a part of.

Conquering Fear

Fear And Desire

Pretty much everything you do is driven by one of two things: fear or desire. Either you desire the beautiful woman, so you will talk to her and try to flirt with her. Or you are afraid of her public rejection, so you will continue to sit with your friends and nurse your Vodka & coke while laughing at each guy who attempts to approach her (until one of them eventually gets a conversation going with her and they leave the bar together 30 minutes later).

Fear or desire drive your decisions and your actions - they're both extremely powerful emotions and both extremely useful in life.

Fear is what keeps you alive on the battlefield. Desire is what brings your victory on the battlefield. When you give in to either emotion, you're a slave to your subconscious, by your instinctual self.

Not a bad thing if running head-first into a shield wall is likely to get you killed. But what about that 5% chance that your axe will land true and crush the skulls of 3 enemies in one swing, spurring fire into the bellies of your brothers behind you and ultimately creating a momentum that ends in the victory of the entire day?

Sometimes listening to your fear isn't the best choice. OR more to the point, it's the safest choice but not the most opportunist choice. Taking a risk on fear can bring your desires closer.

Do you desire to be a King? Do you desire to expand your territory? Do you want to marry the Jarls dötter?

Or do you simply desire to get promoted to Senior Team Leader of Accounts EMEA?

If you are going to achieve any of these things, you're going to need to take risks. You're going to feel fear.

Mortal danger is a fear that most modern men will not have to experience. The fear of death is something you rarely come into contact with (unless you're unfortunate enough to be involved in a crime or accident).

In every day modern life, fears decide and dictate your actions, costing you valuable opportunities and experiences and robbing you of your desires.

Fear has a purpose, to keep us alive. But almost every other fear is wasted. The fear of being rejected by a girl, the fear of failing at an entrepreneurial endeavor, the fear of screwing up a job interview… these fears provide you with no practical benefit. They exist only to hold you back from opportunity and from the chances maybe working out in your favor.

You have zero chance of getting the job if you don't go to the interview. You have some chance of getting the job if you overcome the fear and attend the interview.

So what purpose does fear have in this sense? Will the humiliation of failure really be so crippling to your status in the tribe that you will need to leave the village? Will the shame of your wife really be so extreme that she no longer wishes to produce offspring with you?

When you allow fear to control you and prevent you from chasing your desires, you're listening to outdated biological triggers.

When you learn to become a Viking and dive head first into a shield wall, embracing but throwing aside all fears, you'll start opening yourself to more opportunities and be able to achieve more of your desires.

Identify Your Fears

If you're are going to learn to conquer fear, and be able to show bravery next time you're confronted with fear, you need to learn how to identify and eliminate your current fears.

We all have irrational fears that control us: the fear of spiders, the fear of heights, the fear of ginger people. These fears are the craziest as you can't even rationalize them with any mild risk to yourself, never mind any mortal risk.

You need to honestly list (yes, write an actual list on paper or on your phone) all of your irrational fears. These fears might not be holding you back form many opportunities, but they're making you feel that it's okay to be a slave to your fears. It isn't.

Once you've identified your irrational fears, you need to identify your long-standing rational fears. These are things that you've just always been nervous or afraid of.

Examples might be approaching women, or approaching groups of women, or driving your car alone, or speaking to your manager, or making eye contact with your father... Each of these fears may have a rational root cause and will almost definitely be holding you back from opportunities.

Once you've listed these long-standing fears, make a new section for your most recent fears. What were you afraid of doing yesterday? What about the upcoming day scares you? These fears will likely be much milder in nature, for example, yesterday you were afraid to confront the woman who cut in front of you in the shopping mall line, or you were afraid to correct the waiter who charged you $3 too much by mistake, or you might be nervous about your Tinder date tonight.

Once you've made a list of these 3 major types of fear in your life, you've taken the first step in conquering your fears!

Identifying and admitting to ourselves what actually makes us afraid is a powerful tool. It allows you to accept that you're still a man even though you have these fears. It allows you to accept them and be conscious of them, lifting the fear out of your subconscious where it has more control over you.

The Cost Of Fear

With your fears identified and listed, you need to start analyzing the cost of these fears on your life. Once you know the cost of these fears and how much opportunity they're taking from you, you can get one step closer to realizing how bad these fears are and gaining more motivation to conquer them.

Go back to your list, and next to each of your fears write a number between 1-10 to rank how much each fear is costing you in opportunities and experiences.

- 1 means the fear isn't really costing you anything
- 10 means the fear is robbing you of rich life experiences

These cost rankings aren't the ultimate factor in deciding whether a fear needs to be conquered. As I mentioned earlier, all fears should be conquered. Fear cannot be allowed to control you and you cannot afford to feed any of your fears, no matter how small they are.

However, some of the most difficult and scary fears are the ones that cost us the most opportunity in life.

For example, I had a huge fear of flying. I'd never flown as a child or teenager and the very thought of the whole experience petrified me. I remember turning down multiple "Boys Holidays" abroad and even free holidays with girlfriend's families because I couldn't bring myself to fly.

It was the whole experience - the stress and anxiety of timing the flights and transfers, the stress of the crowds at the airport, the security checks, the turbulence I'd heard about... For years this fear crippled my experiences until one day one of my closest brothers offered me an all expenses paid business trip to USA and Canada. He knew my situation and pretty much held my hand for the entire experience (I'm 22 at this point). By the end of the trip, I felt like such a fool.

I'd missed so many amazing experiences in my life because I'd held this (pretty irrational) fear of traveling via Airport and fear of flying. The cost to my happiness and experiences had been huge!

The cost of fear can be huge and knowing what awaits you as a reward for conquering that fear can be a great motivator.

Desensitizing Yourself To Fear

The only way to conquer some fears is through desensitization - regularly exposing yourself to that fear (building up the intensity in increments each time) until you realize the fear no longer bothers you.

This is a popular psychological treatment in modern therapy, and one the Vikings practiced regularly also.

When a Viking warrior stood in the shield wall, facing a wall of equally skilled, equally ruthless and equally savage enemies, the likelihood of taking a short sword to the gut was extremely high. However, by the time a Viking warrior reached 18 or 19 years old, he had likely stood in this exact situation 5 or 6 times (Viking boys were taking on local skirmishes from the age of 13).

This repeated exposure to mortal danger meant that the Viking warrior was no longer entirely crippled by this fear. Of course, the fear doesn't go away... but your body learns to handle it in a different way.

Just as your Viking brothers stood in the shield wall again and again until they no longer shit themselves, you too need to regularly expose yourself to your fears to become desensitized to them.

If you're afraid of spiders, visit an exotic pet shop. Explain to the store assistant that you have a fear of spiders and you would like to slowly desensitize yourself to them. I've owned a few exotic pets in my time and I can tell you that 100% of guys who work in these shops absolutely love their job, and they love their animals, and will be all too happy to help you to remove your fear of them.

I started by simply viewing the animals through the plastic containers (and slowly learned to control my less-than-masculine screams of surprise when they moved onto the glass)! Then I started asking the guy to remove the lids and take one out, and I would just stand near him while he held it. This stage took a long time for me, probably around 10 visits over the course of a few weeks. Then the man started encouraging the spiders and lizards and creepy crawlies to walk onto my hand, just for a few seconds, then he would take them back.

After a few months, the sweats and racing heart had gone. I wouldn't say I built a love of spiders and scorpions, but I did end up buying a pet lizard (who I fed living creepy crawlies and baby spiders to multiple times a day, by hand, without issue).

Desensitizing myself to my fear of spiders and creepy insects didn't directly increase the amount of opportunities and experiences available to me in life, but it did help me to realize that irrational fears can be conquered, and with each fear, irrational or rational, I erased from my list, the stronger and braver I became when I approached my next fear.

––––––

I'm coming back to this chapter to add another example that recently happened with a coaching client.

Let's call this guy Dave. Dave has many things in his life that he'd like to work on as part of his Modern Viking transformation, but one of the most surprising is his massive anxiety and low-self esteem in his day job when it comes to authoritative colleagues.

Dave is a large guy, extremely good looking and fairly well dressed. He looks "alpha" on the surface. He looks like he could be the Manager or even CEO of his company.

But he's a regular team member (the lowest position in his company), his body language is (or was) extremely sullen and weak, and he regularly gets walked all over by his colleagues.

From the stories Dave told me, I didn't think his colleagues were bad people. They were just taking advantage of Dave's attitude and fears to make their jobs easier. Dave, a fully grown man in his 30's with a wife and children, was literally petrified at the thought of talking to the manager of his department. He had taken sick days before on days when he had his Performance Review because the anxiety of sitting face to face with his boss was too crippling.

Dave was at the point of resigning from his (pretty well paid) job because he thought that all of the guys there didn't like him and he would always be stuck at the bottom, getting walked over by all of the other men and women he worked with.

I knew that the best approach for Dave would be a gradual desensitization to his perception of authority in his company. I suspected that his fears were mostly irrational and they were about to cost him his job, plus his happiness and overall positive energy levels.

We started with Dave slowly making more conversations with his peers - other team members on the same level as him. We practiced the simple act of saying *"Hello"* and making eye contact in the mornings, and he made a very deliberate effort to walk past the desks of his team leader, and then later his manager, saying *"Good Morning"* each time. We focused on making the simple greeting strong, with strong and confident body language and eye contact, and smiling!

After a few weeks, Dave started to make idle conversation whenever his path crossed with colleagues who were more senior than him (I usually despise idle conversation but in this case, it was effective). By this point he was already making comfortable conversations with the other team members who held the same authority level as him.

Last week, Dave emailed me to tell me he went to drinks on Friday afternoon with the whole team! He told me that he was relaxed around both his colleagues and the senior managers who attended.

He realized that his fears were irrational - they were extremely nice guys and they liked him too, they just hadn't been able to find out anything about him because he was also so quiet and nervous.

Dave is now also taking Boxing lessons with a senior colleague in another department - something he would never have been able to bring himself to do before he started practicing desensitizing himself to his fear of authoritative people in his company. I'm confident it will only be a matter of months before he starts getting recognized for his achievements in the company and gets promoted. But more importantly, he's happy and the huge source of negativity in his day has gone. He conquered his fears and he'll be better equipped to conquer future fears that he needs to face.

The Fear Of Rejection

One of the most common fears that men face, particularly in their teens and 20's, is the fear of rejection - particularly the fear of rejection from women.

This fear isn't entirely irrational. Socially speaking, if you approached a woman in the tribe and she rejected you, then you may look weaker to the other men in the tribe. Other women may think that they also should reject you, particularly if they would like to be seen as higher status like the woman who rejected you. This one rejection from this woman could have knock-on effects within the whole tribe and seriously damage your status and reputation (and therefore ability to fuck lots of women and make lots of offspring)!

However... we don't live in small tribes of 100 people anymore. We live in cities of millions of people. While a reputation does follow us, particularly with social media, we no longer run the risk of lowering our status to a crippling low because one woman in a bar rejected us.

To conquer this fear, you need to take two approaches:

1. You need to desensitize yourself to it through regular practice
2. You need to rationally and consciously consider the real risks and consequences of it

Whether you're trying to deal with the fear of rejection from women, or rejection from job offers, or rejection of your creative work, the process to conquer it is the same.

You need to simply get out there and do it, again and again.

Approaching women is scary... for the first 10. The next 25 are less scary. The next 50 are enjoyable and the next 100 are positively exhilarating! I'm not a huge fan of PUA philosophy and it's not what this book is about, but one area where the guys have it right is that when you approach women again, and again, and again, you eventually conquer your fear.

I have a girl friend who was absolutely stone cold petrified of applying for jobs because of the fear of rejection. She had only ever applied for a handful of jobs in her life and they were always jobs that she knew she would get - because she was overqualified and the pay was so low that they probably had only a handful of applicants. This fear was costing her from getting a really great job.

As a friend, I slowly made her realize she needed to apply to lots of jobs. One day we applied to 5. The next we applied to 10. The next week, she applied to nearly 25 jobs a day! Sure enough, she received 90% rejection emails or simply no reply. We were applying to some seriously moonshot jobs! But some of them started to come back with interview offers... and now she works in an amazing company, with an amazing culture, in central London in beautiful posh offices, for nearly 4x her original salary. And the great thing is, everyone who works there had to go through the same crazy application processes that only the most fearless and brave people would do, so now all of her colleagues are simply awesome people.

What was it that allowed her to apply to nearly 200 jobs after spending years only every applying to 2 or 3 jobs whenever she wanted to move job?

It was her realization that there were no negative consequences from a rejection.

If a company doesn't want to hire you, they don't call up your current employer and say *"Hey you should know, this person wants to quit!"* and even in the rare circumstances that does happen, do you know what happens 99% of the time? Your current employer comes and offers you a pay rise!

If they ignore your application (the most irritating), it really doesn't harm you. You're not any worse off than before you applied. Maybe you spent a few minutes or half an hour on that application, but that time was also an investment in yourself - connecting to your strengths and weaknesses and whatever other questions they asked you in the application.

No matter what the rejection, you need to rationalize the real life consequences and costs of the rejection. As with all your Mindset work, you need to move the impulsive thoughts from your subconscious into your conscious so that you can feed the correct emotions and conquer the negative emotions that we don't want.

When you're next about to do something that exposes you and makes you vulnerable to the fear of rejection, literally say to yourself "What's the worst that can happen if I get rejected?". Say this aloud. Say it in your head. Repeat it 10 times. And make sure your friends are onboard with it too - they need to be compounding your positive response to rejection, not encouraging a negative response.

For example, banter among brothers is a serious component to bonding. But when you walk back over to your table after a cute girl has just rejected you, you need to know that your brothers are going to say *"Oh well, so what. This bar is full of cute girls!"*. As we'll discuss in the third part to this book, building the right Tribe around you is a crucial component of becoming a Modern Viking!

The Fear Of Failure

Similar to the fear of rejection, a common fear crippling many is the fear of failure. Rather than social rejection and failing to receive validation, the fear of failure is more material in nature.

The fear of failure is one of the biggest opportunity-costing fears you will face - it's what holds you back from publishing the book that's been inside you for years, it's what holds you back from quitting your job to launch that new startup, it's what holds you back from entering the upcoming inter-club tournament at your Jujitsu gym.

The fear of failure is usually costing you from the opportunity to acquire significant financial or emotional reward. It's a fear I can connect with very intimately - as an entrepreneur who has launched 7 companies, many of them with significant outside investors and my most recent with hundreds of thousands of dollars of other people's money.

In my opinion, conquering the fear of failure is 98% of the difference between entrepreneurs and non-entrepreneurs. Everything else is just skills and connections that can be gained or made. But when you can conquer your fear of failure, you become more powerful and brave than most people in the world and can dive into a new enterprise, company or project without worrying about the consequences.

Conquering your fear of failure, no matter what the scale of the project is, does not mean you ignore the consequences. Just as with conquering your other fears, it's an exercise in gaining perspective and in moving those fears from your subconscious, where they can control you, to your subconscious.

If you write an 80,000 word book and then sell 50 copies, so what? What's the worst thing about this? Embarrassment from friends? Financial costs? Wasted time?

Friends who don't support your projects, successful or otherwise, are not friends.

The financial costs from most projects can often be minimized, and I would say never risk money that you aren't prepared to lose.

And any time spent producing something like a book should not be seen as investment sunk into a product, but rather an education process.

People pay $10,000 to $50,000 to complete a degree on a topic they are interested in. They pay a University a huge sum of money so that they can research and write a large thesis (basically a book) and then senior lecturers at that university can tell them if the thesis was good or not. Yes, that's right, people pay thousands and thousands to basically write a book, because the process of researching and writing that book is an investment into their own education.

So the alternative, is that you spend no money. You research and write that book. And then maybe some people will pay you money to read it, or maybe not. But at the end of the day, you gained all of the education and experience in the writing process. Maybe no-one will call you a "Dr" afterwards but titles can be earned in other ways if that's your thing!

The fear of failure usually has very minimal consequences, or consequences that can be minimized, when you really dig into them. Once you rationalize and start to conquer these consequences of failure, and particularly weigh these up against the potential rewards, you'll be able to make every fear of failure your bitch!

Turning Fear Into Excitement

One of the greatest feelings about conquering your fears is when the emotional response of fear starts changing into a response of excitement. After all, both fear and excitement are based on adrenaline. The difference is your Mindset to that response and whether you turn that moment into a positive or a negative one.

Returning to my earlier example of my fear of flying... now I get incredibly excited about the whole process! I create an exciting game out of catching my flight, I get excited by how cute the hostesses are going to be, I get excited during the turbulence, I feel a rush and a buzz when I arrive at my destination and I can look around and see how happy and excited everyone is!

When you start turning your fears into excitement, you've gone beyond simply conquering fears and you've started to make those fears your bitch! You'll be the Viking who doesn't just stand firm against his enemies, but rushes in with your axe swinging and a crazy smile on your face!

Many situations and scenarios that cause you to be afraid are potentially very rewarding and exciting in and of themselves, not just in their consequences or outcomes.

For example, conquering your fear of approaching women in bars means that you'll open yourself to the very exciting prospect of having sex with a beautiful woman! But if you learn to turn the experience of approaching women itself into something exciting, then you'll be able to enjoy the entire experience. Even if the encounter doesn't go any further into a date or sex, you'll be able to take enjoyment from simply enjoying her company and from the challenge of flirting with her.

Stepping into a boxing ring (or any other competitive martial art) is extremely frightening. Both before and after my first ever Kickboxing match, I remember emptying my guts for so long that I couldn't believe I had any internal organs left!

I felt light headed, I felt scared and I felt like I didn't want to be there.

But after the second, the third, the tenth match, I started to feel a buzz, an excitement, a genuine passion for the fights! I wanted to rush in and punch the guy in the face and get kicked in the face and just generally throw myself in and enjoy the experience! Conquering this fear wasn't just about opening myself up to the opportunity to win the National Heavyweight Championship, it was about being able to enjoy every fight that stood between me and that title.

As you work through your list and you start to desensitize yourself to each fear, to start conquering them one by one and to start opening yourself to the opportunities that await you for defeating them, you should also start to think about how to make the process of conquering those fears genuinely exciting.

Instead of conquering your fear of water by attending swimming classes, why not join a surfing school? Instead of conquering your fear of public speaking by attending a business speaking workshop, why not join a stand up comedy club? Instead of getting over your fear of violence by taking self defense classes, join an MMA gym and enter into amateur tournaments!

Remember, you don't need to measure your 'success' in any of these activities by their own grading systems (catching the biggest wave, getting the whole room in laughter, winning the tournament...etc) For you, the success is in being able to enjoy something that used to make you scared. The success is in finding excitement where there used to only be fear.

Comfort Zones

As you begin to conquer your fears, you will notice your list of fears starting to become very short. When your list starts to run out, when you've started to conquer most of the fears that used to rule your life, you run the risk of approaching a very dangerous place - your comfort zone.

This is the place of stagnation for a Modern Viking. You're not getting any stronger, you're not improving, you're not opening your life to more potentially awesome experiences and rewards.

When you recognize you're getting close to a comfort zone phase, it's very hard to want to change. After months or maybe even years of feeling unhappy, of low confidence and low self-esteem, you finally feel like "the man". Like a warrior. You can approach women, you can talk to your boss as an equal, you aren't afraid of driving anymore. It's very easy and very tempting to stay in this place of "being okay".

And thats where a lot of middle-aged men end up.

Things are okay, they aren't bad enough to complain, there's no need to take any new risks, to push yourself beyond your current position.

But thats where the so called "mid-life crisis" starts. Your life improved at a rapid pace in your 20's and 30's and then when you seemingly conquered all of the things you wanted to change and improve, you stopped and got comfortable.

But regardless of your age or stage in your Modern Viking journey, no matter how great things might seem in your life, you cannot allow yourself to get comfortable!

Comfort zones aren't necessarily, in fact rarely, financial. Sure your job could probably be better or your house bigger, but think beyond that. If you get to the point where you've stopped pushing yourself, then it means you've gotten to a point where you aren't pushing for excitement anymore. You aren't throwing yourself against situations that are frightening, and therefore potentially new exciting experiences.

You might have won "the game" by getting a beautiful girlfriend who has become your best friend. But if you fall into a comfort zone and forget what it means to be bold and confident in social situations, then you run the risk of appearing stagnant or boring to her. Love is very forgiving, but don't forget the man you were when you first charmed her.

You might feel like "the top dog" in your job, but if you lose that hunger for self development, attending conferences and completing extra courses, you'll stop being that strong and fearless guy who came up through the ranks. You'll stagnate, and eventually become irrelevant.

While you want to learn to conquer your fears, you don't ever want to run out of fears to work on. You need to constantly push yourself to conquer new experiences, push yourself harder and push yourself beyond your comfort zone. Your comfort zone is a dynamic and constantly evolving concept, and the most masculine quality you could demonstrate over the years is one of constantly improving, of always becoming better, stronger, braver.

Stop Being Mr Nice Guy

Too many men think that being the gentlemen is always the right solution. Sacrifice your desires for the greater good. Be polite. Avoid unnecessary confrontation.

The problem with being a nice guy, is you rarely get what you want.

But when you embrace an assertive mindset and start acting like an assertive Viking, you can start getting the things you actually desire.

Modern Vikings know that kingdoms and plunder are not awarded to the Nice Guys. Sometimes you need to pickup your axe and shield and stand firm for what you want. You need to have a clear idea of your ambition and your desires, and then be prepared to defend those desires against anyone who challenges them!

Vikings Know What They Want

Being assertive doesn't mean going to battle, necessarily. It means knowing what's worth going to battle for.

An assertive Viking is clear about what he wants. He's sure of his desires and not afraid to express them.

When you start showing this conviction in your desires, and you have a reason to go to battle (if needed), you stop avoiding confrontation - because you know the battle is worth it.

If you're a nice guy, you never stand in the shield wall because you don't even know why you'd be standing there. You aren't sure if you really want to be king or if you want to be the best damn farmer ever. You're not sure if you want to be a forester or a fisherman. You aren't sure if you want to bed Helga or Lagartha tonight.

Nice guys don't get what they want because they aren't sure what they want. A Modern Viking knows his desires and knows they're worth fighting for.

Fighting With The Shield Versus Fighting With The Axe

Often when you express your desires, when you make it known what it is that you want, other people are going to challenge you.

They're going to challenge you because they spot weakness or because your desires will be at the expense of theirs. Sometimes people challenge your assertiveness just because they're fuckwits.

However, one of the most important lessons you need to learn as a Viking, is how to defend your desires and fight for them.

Because a Viking doesn't show his assertiveness with the axe - he uses the shield. Here's the thing - when you use the axe to attack the other person, you're no longer being assertive - you're being aggressive.

Knowing how to hold your shield with a strong arm, pushing back when challenged but always standing firm, is the key to being assertive.

When you attack with the axe, it tends to make other people uncomfortable. They get defensive and guarded themselves, they start lashing out with their own axe. They realize they need to take you down or risk being taken down.

In most situations, being aggressive won't just not get you what you desire, but it will make the situation worse and you could end up with even less.

Why You Can't Just Berserk Every Situation

Life would be simpler if you could dive into every problem with axe swinging. Whenever you want something, you could pull out the axe and swing it into those blocking your way.

When you want the special daytime menu but it's already gone past 5pm, it would be great if a few swings of your axe would cut down the waiter and force the manager to still honor the deal.

When your girlfriend wants to watch the cheesy romantic movie instead of the latest Marvel movie, it would be fantastic if a swift brandishing of your axe had her cowering in fear as she obediently carries your popcorn into the latest Thor vs. Hulk cinematic massacre.

When your working group unanimously decides to go with David's social media strategy over yours, life would be magical if a few overhead swings of your axe would leave only the bloodied and disemboweled corpse of David as a lasting reminder of his inferior presentation.

Unfortunately, Modern Vikings need to know when situations call for the axe, and when they call for the shield. When it's time to be assertive and stand for what you want, defending and pushing back, but respecting your opponents ground too.

How To Fight For What You Want, With Only A Shield

When you want something and you're expecting to have to fight for it, knowing how to fight with only your shield is an important skill that every Modern Viking needs to learn.

Vikings were famous for their well rehearsed and trained shield tactics in battle. Working as a unit, the Viking shield wall was a formidable but forgotten battle tactic (of course, Roman soldiers had been using a variety of precise shield formations over 1,000 years before the Vikings invaded England and northern Europe). While the strength of the shield wall came from the brotherhood and trust of Viking brothers working together, it was only made possible by each Viking becoming as intimately familiar with his shield as a tool on the battlefield as he was his axe or sword.

Often with a strong iron butt in the centre, a thick wooden shield would not only protect a viking from deathly blows, but it could be used to push back into the enemy or even attack (using the iron butt) if needed.

When it comes to being a Modern Viking, your shield is your conviction and your solid sense of self-worth and confidence. It's your passion for your desires. It's your ability to express those desires in a solid and definitive tone that causes your potential opponents to think twice before trying to challenge you.

An assertive Modern Viking is able to fight for what he wants without needing to attack anyone.

How To Express Yourself Assertively

Expressing yourself in an assertive way is the best way to avoid the need to defend your desires at all.

- Using short and concise sentences
- Using definitive language
- Avoid justification or apologies
- Maintaining eye contact
- Speaking clearly and with a confident tonality

By speaking in short, concise and clear sentences, you leave nothing open to interpretation or misunderstanding. And by using definitive language like *"it is"* instead of *"it might be"*, you leave no holes or weak spots that other people could exploit and second-guess.

Strong and confident body language ensures that your desires are delivered correctly, and people can see that you're carrying them with conviction. When you're timid and nervous about expressing yourself, people will just ignore you and aggressive people will dominate you.

Picking Out Weakness In The Shield Wall

Common signs of people who are not being assertive and who's assertiveness will immediately be challenged:

- Using unsure language such as "maybe" and "perhaps"
- Using way too many words to express themselves
- Not maintaining eye contact
- Trailing off at the end of sentences
- Having weak and unsure tonality
- Being overly courteous, i.e. *"If it isn't too much of a bother…"*
- Worrying too much about other people's desires

Assertive Vikings In The Workplace

When you want to take your Modern viking assertiveness to the workplace, there are a few additional techniques that will help to ensure your desires are understood and known, whilst avoiding conflict and affecting the professionalism.

Whenever you ask something of your colleagues, and particularly of people who you manage, many people are too quick to justify or even apologize for their requests.

"I'm sorry Dave, but do you mind getting those reports to me today?"

"I'm sorry Sarah but I needed those designs to me on Friday because of the printers, so if it isn't too much hassle, can you stay an extra 30 minutes to finish them?"

As a manager, but also as a colleague working with your peers, whenever you set a task that you need completing, ensuring it has a clear target with clear deliverables means that everyone knows exactly what you want and by when.

Setting a deadline gives a clear expectation of when it needs to be finished by and with plenty of notice. And presumably, you have a very good reason for that timeline.

However, when you're too quick to justify that timeline to the person, or even worse you apologize for it, you open yourself to being challenged and people will no longer have faith in your assertiveness.

People confuse this with showing empathy and compassion for your colleague. It's possible to empathize and that means allowing them to immediately notify you if they have any problems with the task, something blocking it that you weren't aware of or perhaps they just aren't confident in their ability to deliver it in that time window.

By allowing everyone to feel heard and respected, you're empathizing with your colleague.

But at the end of the day, your job is to get the tasks delivered and you don't need to justify or apologize for that. Your colleague doesn't need to know the reason why you need it by Tuesday, they just need to have faith and belief that you wouldn't ask for it by Tuesday if you didn't have a good reason. And that comes with being assertive and having conviction.

Make sure to build a reputation at work of holding people accountable to their deadlines, especially when they miss them, and ensure that people know not to try last minute excuses or complaints with their Modern Viking manager. Your job at work is not to be peoples friends or to be the nice guy - it's to be the guy who gets shit done.

Bending The Knee

The exception to being assertive in the workplace is if you're the guy being told what to do by your assertive Modern Viking manager. In this situation, do you suddenly have to stop being a Modern Viking yourself, and become a Mr Nice Guy?

Of course not!

Viking Jarls (Norse Earls, Lords) ruled their own territory - they had soldiers, they collected tax and they enforced the laws. But they also answered to a King (a Viking King was usually a very successful Jarl who declared himself King and nearby Jarls chose to accept his rule).

A Jarl was a powerful warlord in his own right - he could be assertive in expressing his desires to his own people, to his wife and to his brothers. But he also needed to know when to serve his king.

Even the famous Viking Rollo, first Duke of Normandy, once said *"never will I bend my knee before any man"*[16]. But he still accepted the King of France's rule and pledged his fealty to follow orders if they were given!

As long as you feel respected, and the person asking something of you is not aggressive or overly dominant, there is nothing "not Viking" about going along with their request. As long as you have the opportunity to make yourself heard and everyone in the situation feels comfortable, doing as your asked is just a part of life. It's part of the system and it's how shit gets done.

Be More Assertive In 3 Steps

To be more assertive, you can follow 3 simple rules:

1. Shut up and think about what you actually want and desire from the situation first

2. Say what you want with as few words as possible, with definitive language and confident body language

3. Have conviction in your decision if it's challenged and be prepared to fight with the shield!

---

[16] John Hayward (2015), *Northmen.* https://books.google.com/books?isbn=1781855226

Only The Gods Know

"The unwise man is awake all night worries over and again. When morning rises he is restless still, his burden as before."

- The Havamal

Vikings were blessed with a freedom from worry and anxiety because of their mindset on fate. Emboldened by their religious beliefs and driven by a desire to enjoy the theatre of life, they were able to release themselves from the stress and unhappiness of worrying over choices because a large part of their destiny was already being written by someone else.

Because the Vikings believed that the fate/destiny, or urðr, of every man was already decided (in a fairly solid but still somewhat malleable way).

They believed that the 3 Norns (divine beings) sat beneath the roots of Yggdrasil, the tree of life. There, they weaved the threads of each man's life. Urðr (fate), Verðandi (present) and Skuld (future) would record the knowledge and destiny of every man and God. They saw everything that had passed and was currently happening, everything that could come to pass and everything that would come to pass.

They and they alone held the knowledge of the world and the knowledge of destiny.

Well, until Odin half killed himself to earn some of that knowledge too!

When a Viking charged into the enemy's shield wall, or he decided whether to join a Viking campaign to England or to Frankia, he knew that he needn't worry about making the incorrect choice. There was no correct or incorrect choice - only the Gods knew for sure. So his only role in life was to throw himself at the situation with all that he had, all that his skills and training allowed him to, and to enjoy the journey of life in this world before his journey would take him to Valhalla.

Vikings embraced the idea that a man can only know so much about his destiny, and the possibilities of each branch of choice he made. He embraced that he held a measure of free will over his destiny, but he also accepted that the Gods forged part of his fate too. His best choice was to make the very best of every story that the Norns weaved into his life.

You Are Prone To Assume The Worst

You are naturally prone to worry about the worst case situation. For ancient man crossing an ocean, he was more likely to fear the possibility of a storm sinking his ship than he was to worry that the salted pork would be unpleasant to eat. When you fly on a plane today, you are more likely to fear the plane exploding in mid air and crashing than you are to fear getting seated next to a really fat guy.

Your mind is terrible at running to the worst case scenario all the time, and you tend to amplify the likelihood of those terrible possibilities so much so that you become racked with worry. This worry can consume you and plant all kinds of negative emotions in your day.

Every time I started a new company and I took other people's money, my mind's immediate reaction was to begin to worry about losing every cent of that investment. Within seconds I'm running the news headlines through my minds eye, the New York Times declaring "Failed Entrepreneur Blows $10 million in 6 Months" and my parents giving me a phone call to let me know how disappointed they are in me. Within a few more minutes, my heart is fighting it's way out of my chest and I'm physically fearful and sick from worry.

Despite the fact that these absolutely horrible scenarios are very unlikely (failing in business is very likely, but failing so spectacularly rarely happens) it doesn't stop my mind from trying to respond with this mindset.

However, learning to catch yourself before you fall into these deep worry spells is crucial for your long term happiness and also your ability to make sound decisions. Which is important, because the situations that cause us the most worry are usually the situations that require us to be at our absolute sharpest.

Be mindful that an untrained mind will always fall to the worst case scenario - so how do you learn to deal with this and pull yourself back? How did the Vikings religious beliefs free them from worry? How do I steam head-first into startups with other people's investment without staying awake all night?

Considering The Real Worst Case Outcome

When we dive into these deepest depths of worry and we consider all of the terrible things that might happen, we actually are capable of imaging scenarios at are nearly impossible. We imagine worst case scenarios that are even worse than the worst.

If I fail at a startup, the New York Times is almost definitely not going to write about my failure. My Dad is almost definitely not going to tell me he's disappointed in me. A kitten is almost definitely not going to die.

So what is the likely worst case scenario?

When you apply for a job, is it really likely that by the end of the interview, all 5 people on the panel will be pointing and laughing at you because you projectile vomited from nerves, coating the assistant, who's transcribing the conversation, in chunks of your breakfast burrito?

When you consider approaching a group of women in a bar, is it really likely that in the 16 steps it takes you to get over to them, you are going to trip over the carpet, grabbing a handful of the bouncers junk on the way down as your thrash wildly for balance, and then hit the floor so hard that you knock yourself out and then piss your pants in your moments of blackout sleep?

When worry strikes before a situation, you need to calmly and rationally consider the realistic worst case scenario. It still might not be pretty, but it's probably not as bad as your irrational brain would have you believe.

Accepting The Worst Case

Once you've become aware of the worst case scenario, you need to visualize yourself in that scenario. Put yourself there. Imagine it has happened, and come to terms with the fact.

Come to terms with the fact that your ship might crash on rocks. Come to terms with the fact that half of your boats may be lost in a storm. Come to terms with the fact that the Parisians may actually know how to defend their city from your horde of savage Viking warriors.

Be aware of how you would feel, how you would be, in that moment. Allow the feelings of that moment (not after that moment, just the moment itself) to set in.

And now breathe. Take a few breaths. Probably doesn't feel as bad as you expected, right?

Analysis Paralysis

The initial fear from the possibility of worst case scenarios causes us to be apprehensive about making any decision. You trick yourself into believing that until you make a decision, the worst case scenario can't happen yet. You try to delay the inevitable.

But time is cyclic and the waters from the tree of life will keep flowing regardless of whether you choose to partake in the story. What this means is that you can stand still, paralyzed by the inability and fear of making a decision, for so long that the situation becomes worse or passes you by all together.

This manifests moreso than ever in the workplace, particularly if you're in any management position. One of the earliest skills I learned when managing a team of employees at just 18 was that the damage of making no decision far outweighed the potential damage of making the wrong decision. My employees, equally as junior as me, would come to me to make a call: this technology or that one? This quote or that quote? Ship this client's project first or that client?

The time wasted by stalling on decisions is time not invested into executing on your decision.

As I grew older, I learned to forget the very concept of a wrong decision all together. There was only one type of choice, and that was the correct choice, made to the best of my ability with everything available to me at that time.

As long as I followed a thorough analysis of all of the facts available to me at the time, experience had taught me that the only wrong decision was making no decision.

Trying To Improve The Worst Case

Once you've freed yourself from the anxiety of making a choice, you've accepted that at least some choice needs to be made, and you've already created a boundary limit of the absolute worst case scenario, then you can begin to work on making that worst case outcome better.

Unfortunately as a Viking, you don't have much control over the weather. But what if you did lose half of your boats before landing ashore, how could you make that situation better?

Well, you could ensure that the archers are evenly distributed across the fleet. You could ensure that no more than 1 Jarl or leader travels in each boat. Likewise, you could evenly distribute the food rations for the campaign across the fleet. Perhaps also instruct men to ensure they do not wear their armor while sailing to give each man at least a slim chance of swimming to safety.

In your life, you could both reduce the likelihood of your worst case scenario happening, or you could implement tactics to lessen the impact of the worst case scenario.

To revisit our earlier examples, you could try to not eat much food before you interview and at the slightest feeling of nausea, you could excuse yourself to the bathroom. Before approaching the woman in the bar, you could ensure to take extra care with walking across the bar and you could maybe visit the bathroom first to make sure you aren't going to piss your pants as you hit the floor!

Both silly examples but designed to illustrate a point - fate is never as cruel to us as we worry about.

Embrace Your Destiny And Reduce Worry In 3 Steps

1. Consider the realistic worst case scenario
2. Visualize yourself in that worst case scenario and accept the emotions and consequences of that absolute worst case
3. Now begin to implement changes to make that worst case scenario less likely to happen, and to lessen the impact of it if it does

Now Go Viking!

"One's back is vulnerable, unless one has a brother."

Ber er hver að baki nema sér bróður eigi.

- The Saga of Grettir, chapter 82

Brotherhood

In Viking culture, brotherhood was extremely important. Your brothers protected your flank in the shield wall, they protected your head, they pulled you back during danger and they gave you the strength to push forward during times of fear.

To a Modern Viking, the importance of Brotherhood is no different.

Whether you're trying to find the motivation to go to the gym, the confidence to go to a bar and talk to a beautiful girl, or you just want to have a few beers and grill some meat and have a good time feasting, having positive and likeminded men around you is extremely important.

Your brothers can support you on your fitness journey - and the road to a Modern Viking transformation is a long one. I started to put my own story online on Instagram around 9 months ago, but I know that my physical transformation is going to take 5+ years.

To make it easier for Modern Vikings all over the world, I've created Brotherhood, an online community for Modern Vikings to hang out and support each other.

In this peer-to-peer community, Modern Vikings who are serious about their transformation can talk privately and support each other. You can ask each other questions, share stories of what is working and what isn't, and together we can evolve the Modern Viking movement.

Of course, I'm also extremely active in Brotherhood too!

I've also recruited some of the amazing experts who helped me with the research for Modern Viking to answer specific questions - these are people who are my mentors and my inspirations.

In Brotherhood you'll find world bodybuilding champions, military officers, crossfit coaches, nutritionists, male and female psychologists, PUA's, farmers, fisherman, foresters, boxers, MMA fighters… and also lots of regular guys. Accountants, lawyers, stay at home dads.

Brotherhood is about coming together over the values and strength of character that Modern Viking encourages and galvanizes in every man.

Check it out here:

http://liamgooding.com/brotherhood

Build A Tribe

This will probably fail - but such is the way with crazy and ambitious ideas.

I wonder if Modern Vikings all over the world can start bringing together in-person meetups to support each other. These Tribes will be brought together on a single purpose:

"To rediscover male masculinity by revisiting Viking social structures and male bonding"

There are thousands of Modern Vikings reading this book right now who are on their journey alone. You might be really fortunate, you might have a large group of brothers (20+) and have an active social life, with plenty of guys who you can learn from.

We learn from the men around us how to be strong, we challenge ourselves, we push ourselves. We learn how to be funny, we learn how to flirt with women, we learn how to bond and build friendships.

But many guys don't have that. They've been married for 20 years and slowly, their marriage has stripped away their masculinity, their strength, their brotherhood.

But worst of all, marriage strips away friendships.

Guys don't have to be divorced or recently dumped to find themselves in this situation - you could simply be surrounded by weak guys. Guys who wouldn't understand your Modern Viking journey. Guys who make for a poor tribe.

Well, I think it's time we try to build stronger tribes. Stronger clans of brothers who want to improve themselves to become stronger, better men, better brothers, better fathers, better husbands.

Modern Viking Tribes have no religious or political alignment or requirement.

Instead, Tribes judge their members on the strength of their character and the strength of their backs.

Age doesn't matter - tribes have always required men from all ages. The wisdom of the older, the strength of the middle aged, the bravery/foolishness of the young.

Membership should have an entry requirement, an invitation and endorsement by another member at a minimum. But I would also hope that the Tribe founders create some kind of entry test that all members, from founder to newest recruit, should complete. Tribal bonding rituals are a long lost art.

This is entirely voluntary - let's see how this experiment unfolds. Email me on hello@liamgooding.com if you are interested in setting up a local Modern Viking Tribe and I will list all of the available Tribes on the website, along with contact information of the founders.

http://liamgooding.com/tribes

The only requirement is that the Tribe founder is an active member of the Brotherhood membership community and is in contact with myself. This will make it easier to co-ordinate and allow all Tribe founders to share ideas and experiences.

My hope is that by giving Modern Vikings worldwide a 'real world' brotherhood to belong to, we can support even more men on their journey.

Authors Notes

Acknowledgements

I need to thank my best friend Corinne. I promised you we'd be rich and I'd give you the world - I seem to have failed. I gave you everything you wanted, but then I fucked it up and we lost it all. I took you through a crazy journey that would test even the strongest of relationships. Thank you for sticking with me and putting up with me for as long as you did. And thank you for continuing to support me as a loving friend throughout this Modern Viking personal journey. I love you, and I hope that someday, you'll be able to forgive me for turning up one morning with a pet wolf!

Thank you to my Brother and mentor in all things life and business, Jon Gwillim. From wiring me £20,000 in the middle of the night without question, to punching me in the back of the head and almost knocking me out, you've always had a way of being there to push me when I need it, but also knowing when to throw out the safety net when I fall. I'm looking forward to our castle siege wars where I am confident we will both kill each other in a glorious battle to make the bards sing for generations.

To my Brother, Coach James Jones, thank you for answering every and any fitness or nutrition question I had while bringing this book together. Thank you for being my iceberg herding partner and for supporting me on many Viking raids.

Thank you to my Brothers in England: John Munn, Adam Denne, Chris Alcock, Pete Langdown. You've all been long-time friends who have stood with me through the victories and the losses. You've seen me at the top and at the bottom, and you've being my Brothers all the same.

Thank you to Jefferson Mosquera and Kevin Bertolli, my Brothers in San Francisco, for taking that *"weird looking straight British guy"* under your wing and teaching me how to dress, how to love life again and how to embrace my love of bottomless mimosas!

Thank you to the friends I've made traveling Spain - you guys made writing this book far more fun. Thank you to Raffa, Valentin, Yoko, Claire, Warwick, Perrieve, Niall, Keith. While my nomadic life may take me somewhere new, you guys have made this chapter in my life so much more magical.

Also a huge thank you to Giulio Amato and all the team at Beach Cafe, Barcelona (where about 80% of this book was written). You guys know how to keep an amazing vibe and energy which was exactly what I needed to write this book. You also have an amazing talent of knowing exactly when to bring me coffee and food when you could see I'd got lost in my writing! From asking me about todays word count, to telling me to go and have a smoke and take a break on the beach, you are the best hosts a book author could ask for!

Thank you to my family for never judging me as the "odd one out" and for always supporting me with their love. Thank you especially to my Dad, Ian Gooding, who raised me as a single parent and gave me more freedom and independence than any young Viking could ask for. I have no doubt in my mind that he is the reason for my entrepreneurial courage and spirit today.

And finally, thank you to the many, many beautiful women in my past who have helped to shape me into the Modern Viking I am today. Some of you were cruel crazy bitches and you taught me how to be strong, fearless and headstrong. Others of you were loving and beautiful people who taught me how to be vulnerable, compassionate and kind. Whether I knew you for a few hours or a few years, there is a part of you in this book and I'm confident that Modern Viking wouldn't be the same without you.

I'm still searching for my Shield Maiden...

- The End -

Made in the USA
San Bernardino, CA
12 November 2016